CARDIOLOGY
Examination Paper 1
for DM (Cardiology) Students

CARDIOLOGY
Examination Paper 1
for DM (Cardiology) Students

Barun Kumar
MD DM (Cardiology)
Additional Professor and Interventional Cardiologist
Department of Cardiology
All India Institute of Medical Sciences
Rishikesh, Uttarakhand, India

Foreword
Gurpreet S Wander

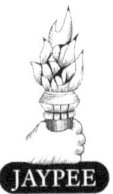

JAYPEE

JAYPEE BROTHERS MEDICAL PUBLISHERS
The Health Sciences Publisher
New Delhi | London

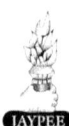 **Jaypee Brothers Medical Publishers (P) Ltd**

Headquarters
Jaypee Brothers Medical Publishers (P) Ltd
EMCA House, 23/23-B
Ansari Road, Daryaganj
New Delhi 110 002, India
Landline: +91-11-23272143,
+91-11-23272703, +91-11-23282021,
+91-11-23245672
Email: jaypee@jaypeebrothers.com

Overseas Office
JP Medical Ltd
83 Victoria Street, London
SW1H 0HW (UK)
Phone: +44 20 3170 8910
Fax: +44 (0)20 3008 6180
Email: info@jpmedpub.com

Corporate Office
Jaypee Brothers Medical Publishers (P) Ltd
4838/24, Ansari Road, Daryaganj
New Delhi 110 002, India
Phone: +91-11-43574357
Fax: +91-11-43574314
Email: jaypee@jaypeebrothers.com

EU GPSR Authorised Representative
LOGOS EUROPE, 9 rue Nicolas Poussin
17000, LA ROCHELLE, France
Phone: +33 (0) 6 67 93 73 78
Email: Contact@logos europe.eu

Website: www.jaypeebrothers.com
Website: www.jaypeedigital.com

© 2024, Jaypee Brothers Medical Publishers

The views and opinions expressed in this book are solely those of the original contributor(s)/author(s) and do not necessarily represent those of editor(s) or publisher of the book.

All rights reserved. No part of this publication may be reproduced, stored or transmitted in any form or by any means, electronic, mechanical, photocopying, recording or otherwise, without the prior permission in writing of the publishers.

All brand names and product names used in this book are trade names, service marks, trademarks or registered trademarks of their respective owners. The publisher is not associated with any product or vendor mentioned in this book.

Medical knowledge and practice change constantly. This book is designed to provide accurate, authoritative information about the subject matter in question. However, readers are advised to check the most current information available on procedures included and check information from the manufacturer of each product to be administered, to verify the recommended dose, formula, method and duration of administration, adverse effects and contraindications. It is the responsibility of the practitioner to take all appropriate safety precautions. Neither the publisher nor the author(s)/editor(s) assume any liability for any injury and/or damage to persons or property arising from or related to use of material in this book.

This book is sold on the understanding that the publisher is not engaged in providing professional medical services. If such advice or services are required, the services of a competent medical professional should be sought.

Every effort has been made where necessary to contact holders of copyright to obtain permission to reproduce copyright material. If any have been inadvertently overlooked, the publisher will be pleased to make the necessary arrangements at the first opportunity.

Inquiries for bulk sales may be solicited at: jaypee@jaypeebrothers.com

Cardiology Examination Paper 1 for DM (Cardiology) Students

First Edition: **2024**

ISBN: 978-93-5696-484-6

Dedicated to

My parents, particularly my father who has provided unwavering support during my preparatory days. It is also dedicated to my teachers, mentors, and family members. This book is specifically intended for students who are diligently pursuing a degree in DM Cardiology.

Foreword

It is a pleasure to write a foreword for this very interesting book *Cardiology Examination Paper 1 for DM (Cardiology) Students*. Dr Barun Kumar, the author of this book has done an excellent work by providing answers to some of the most asked questions in DM Cardiology theory examinations. This is the first book of its kind and will be very useful for students across the country. It covers the topics very precisely and the method of answering is also of very high standard. Besides knowledge of the topic, which is covered, the students will also learn the method of answering these questions.

The author has given very useful references at the end which will make important reading for students who want to learn more about the subject. Answering theory questions is an art which we tend to forget after our graduation since there is emphasis on clinical learning and skill development. This book will fill in this gap in an excellent manner and students can go through it for their exam preparation. The answers are concise, to the point and very well written. When we go back to the standard textbooks, it takes much longer time for covering each topic as compared to this book.

The publisher of the book M/s Jaypee Brothers Medical Publishers (P) Ltd, New Delhi, India is the best medical publisher in the country. It is always a pleasure to read its books since the quality and standards are very high and the publishing is flawless. I wish more such books are brought out by the learned author and the excellent publishers which will cover many other questions that are commonly asked in the DM Cardiology theory examinations. In fact, the students will become better clinicians since their understanding of a subject will improve significantly after going through this book. I have enjoyed reading this book myself and I am sure all those who go through it will find it very informative, simple, and easy to read.

Gurpreet S Wander
DM FACC FAMS
Principal and Professor of Cardiology
Dayanand Medical College and Hospital
Ludhiana, Punjab, India
Chairman
Board of Management
Baba Farid University of Health Sciences
Punjab
Past President
Association of Physicians of India

Preface

Welcome to the comprehensive study guide designed specifically for candidates preparing for the DM Cardiology examination. This book serves as your roadmap to navigate through the intricacies of cardiology, providing a detailed exploration of essential topics crucial for success in your upcoming examination.

Within these pages, you will find in-depth discussions on a wide range of subjects, from congenital heart abnormalities to the dynamic intricacies of cardiovascular physiology. Each chapter is meticulously crafted to offer a thorough understanding of the underlying concepts, supplemented by practical insights and clinical correlations to reinforce your learning.

My goal is to empower you with the knowledge and confidence needed to tackle the exam with proficiency. To aid in your preparation, I have included a variety of question formats, including long-essay questions and answers and short questions and answers, mirroring the structure of the actual examination.

Whether you are embarking on your cardiology journey or seeking to enhance your expertise, this book is your trusted companion. I encourage you to engage actively with the material, leveraging it as a valuable resource to sharpen your skills and deepen your understanding of cardiology.

As you embark on this educational endeavor, remember that perseverance and dedication are key to achieving your goals. I wish you success in your pursuit of excellence in the field of cardiology and trust that this book will serve as a valuable asset in your preparation journey.

Best wishes for your examination success!

Barun Kumar

Acknowledgments

I am sincerely grateful for the support and guidance provided by M/s Jaypee Brothers Medical Publishers (P) Ltd, New Delhi, India throughout this journey. Your invaluable insights and encouragement have been instrumental in helping me refine my ideas and bring them to fruition.

I would also like to extend my gratitude to the entire editorial and production team of M/s Jaypee Brothers Medical Publishers (P) Ltd for their dedication and hard work in ensuring the quality and integrity of the manuscript.

Contents

Paper 1 (Set 1) Long-essay Questions and Answers 1
Short Questions and Answers 4

Paper 1 (Set 2) Long-essay Questions and Answers 15
Short Questions and Answers 18

Paper 1 (Set 3) Long-essay Questions and Answers 31
Short Questions and Answers 34

Paper 1 (Set 4) Long-essay Questions and Answers 44
Short Questions and Answers 47

Index *55*

DM CARDIOLOGY EXAMINATION

Paper 1 (Set 1)

LONG-ESSAY QUESTIONS AND ANSWERS

Q 1. Discuss embryology, pathophysiology of conotruncal abnormalities, and the principles of their management.
(Refer 2014/2019 MUHS, 2009 MGR, 2018 Safdarjung)

Ans. Conotruncal abnormalities encompass a group of congenital heart defects that involve malformations of the outflow tracts of the heart during embryological development. Understanding the embryology, pathophysiology, and principles of management of conotruncal abnormalities is essential for effective clinical management.

- *Embryology:* During embryonic development, the heart forms from the fusion and differentiation of the bilateral cardiogenic plates. The heart tube undergoes looping and septation to form the four-chambered heart with the great vessels. The outflow tracts of the heart, which include the conus arteriosus and truncus arteriosus, give rise to the aorta and pulmonary artery, respectively.
- *Pathophysiology:* Conotruncal abnormalities arise from disruptions in the development of the outflow tracts and are often associated with defects in septation and alignment. Common conotruncal abnormalities include:
  - *Tetralogy of Fallot (TOF):* TOF is characterized by four main features: (1) A ventricular septal defect (VSD), (2) pulmonary stenosis (obstruction of the right ventricular outflow tract), (3) overriding aorta (aorta that straddles the VSD), and (4) right ventricular hypertrophy. These abnormalities result in mixing of oxygenated and deoxygenated blood, leading to cyanosis.
  - *Transposition of the great arteries (TGA):* In TGA, the aorta arises from the right ventricle, and the pulmonary artery arises from the left ventricle, leading to parallel circulation and inadequate oxygenation of blood. This defect typically results in severe cyanosis soon after birth.
  - *Persistent truncus arteriosus:* In this defect, there is failure of septation between the aorta and pulmonary artery, resulting in a single arterial trunk arising from both ventricles. This leads to mixing of oxygenated and deoxygenated blood and subsequent cyanosis.
- *Principles of management:* The management of conotruncal abnormalities typically involves a multidisciplinary approach and may include medical

management, surgical intervention, and long-term follow-up. Principles of management include:
- *Medical stabilization*: Initial management focuses on stabilizing the patient and managing symptoms such as cyanosis, respiratory distress, and heart failure. This may involve supplemental oxygen, intravenous (IV) fluids, and medications to improve cardiac function and reduce pulmonary congestion.
- *Surgical repair*: Definitive treatment for conotruncal abnormalities often requires surgical intervention. The specific surgical procedure depends on the type and severity of the defect but may include repair of the VSD, relief of pulmonary stenosis, arterial switch operation in TGA, or repair of the truncus arteriosus.
- *Timely intervention*: Surgical repair is typically performed in early infancy to optimize outcomes and prevent complications associated with cyanotic heart disease, such as polycythemia, thromboembolism, and developmental delays.
- *Long-term follow-up*: Patients with conotruncal abnormalities require lifelong follow-up with a cardiologist to monitor cardiac function, assess for complications, and optimize medical management. Regular echocardiograms, electrocardiograms, and cardiac imaging may be necessary to monitor for residual defects, valve function, and cardiac function.
- *Genetic counseling*: In cases of syndromic conotruncal abnormalities or family history of congenital heart disease, genetic counseling may be recommended to assess the risk of recurrence in future pregnancies and provide information about inheritance patterns and genetic testing options.

In summary, conotruncal abnormalities result from disruptions in the development of the outflow tracts of the heart during embryological development. Management requires a multidisciplinary approach involving medical stabilization, surgical intervention, and long-term follow-up to optimize outcomes and quality of life for affected individuals. Early diagnosis, timely intervention, and comprehensive care are essential for improving outcomes in patients with conotruncal abnormalities.

Q 2. Discuss accessory pathways of conduction and treatment of related arrhythmias. *(Refer 2019 MUHS)*

Ans. Accessory pathways of conduction, also known as bypass tracts, are abnormal electrical connections between the atria and ventricles of the heart. These pathways bypass the normal conduction system, allowing for rapid conduction of electrical impulses, and predisposing individuals to various types of arrhythmias, most notably Wolff-Parkinson-White (WPW) syndrome. Understanding the anatomy, physiology, and treatment of accessory pathways is crucial for managing arrhythmias associated with these pathways effectively.

- *Anatomy and physiology:* Accessory pathways can be classified based on their location and connection to the atrioventricular (AV) node:
  - *Kent bundles:* These pathways connect the atria and ventricles directly, bypassing the AV node. Kent bundles are characteristic of WPW syndrome.
  - *Mahaim fibers:* These pathways connect the atria and ventricles at the level of the bundle of His or bundle branches. Mahaim fibers are less common than Kent bundles but can also contribute to preexcitation syndromes.

  Accessory pathways allow for rapid conduction of electrical impulses from the atria to the ventricles, bypassing the normal delay at the AV node. This can result in premature activation of the ventricles and predispose individuals to supraventricular tachyarrhythmias, including atrioventricular reentrant tachycardia (AVRT) and atrial fibrillation with rapid ventricular response.

- *Clinical presentation:* Patients with accessory pathways may be asymptomatic or present with symptoms related to arrhythmias, such as palpitations, chest pain, syncope, or sudden cardiac arrest. The presence of characteristic ECG findings, including a short PR interval, delta waves (slurred upstroke of the QRS complex), and widened QRS complexes during tachycardia, can help diagnose WPW syndrome.

- *Treatment of arrhythmias related to accessory pathways:* The treatment of arrhythmias associated with accessory pathways depends on the type of arrhythmia, symptom severity, and underlying cardiac status. Treatment options include:
  - *Observation:* Asymptomatic individuals with WPW pattern on ECG may not require specific treatment but should be monitored regularly for arrhythmias and symptom development.
  - *Acute management of symptomatic arrhythmias:*
    - Vagal maneuvers: Valsalva maneuver or carotid sinus massage can sometimes terminate re-entrant tachyarrhythmias such as AVRT.
    - Adenosine: IV adenosine can be used to terminate paroxysmal supraventricular tachycardia (PSVT) by blocking conduction through the AV node.
    - Electrical cardioversion: Synchronized cardioversion may be necessary for hemodynamically unstable patients with refractory arrhythmias.
  - *Long-term management:*
    - Catheter ablation: Radiofrequency catheter ablation is the treatment of choice for symptomatic accessory pathways. During

the procedure, the abnormal pathway is identified and selectively ablated, interrupting conduction through the pathway.
- Antiarrhythmic medications: Medications such as beta-blockers, calcium channel blockers, or antiarrhythmic drugs (e.g., flecainide and propafenone) may be used to suppress arrhythmias or reduce symptom frequency in patients who are not candidates for or decline catheter ablation.
- Risk assessment and anticoagulation: Patients with WPW syndrome and a history of atrial fibrillation may require anticoagulation to reduce the risk of stroke.

- *Prognosis:* The prognosis for patients with accessory pathways depends on various factors, including the type and location of the pathway, the presence of associated cardiac abnormalities, and the effectiveness of treatment. With appropriate management, including catheter ablation, the majority of patients can achieve resolution of symptoms and normalization of cardiac conduction.

In summary, accessory pathways of conduction are abnormal electrical connections between the atria and ventricles that can predispose individuals to supraventricular tachyarrhythmias. Treatment options include observation, acute management of symptomatic arrhythmias, and long-term management strategies such as catheter ablation and antiarrhythmic medications. Timely intervention and individualized treatment plans are essential for optimizing outcomes in patients with accessory pathway-related arrhythmias.

SHORT QUESTIONS AND ANSWERS

Q 1. Cyanotic spell. *(Refer 2012/2019 MUHS)*

Ans. Cyanotic spell, also known as cyanotic episode or "tet spell," are acute exacerbations of cyanosis (bluish discoloration of the skin and mucous membranes) in infants and young children with congenital heart defects, particularly those with TOF. TOF is a complex congenital heart defect characterized by four main features:

1. *Ventricular septal defect*: A hole in the wall (septum) that separates the right and left ventricles.
2. *Pulmonary stenosis*: Narrowing of the pulmonary valve or pulmonary artery, which restricts blood flow to the lungs.
3. *Overriding aorta*: The aorta is positioned directly over the VSD, allowing oxygen-poor blood from the right ventricle to flow into the aorta and mix with oxygen-rich blood from the left ventricle.

4. *Right ventricular hypertrophy*: Enlargement of the right ventricle due to increased workload.

During a cyanotic spell, several factors contribute to a sudden decrease in systemic arterial oxygen saturation, leading to worsening cyanosis and potentially life-threatening hypoxemia. The exact mechanisms underlying cyanotic spells are not fully understood, but they are believed to involve a combination of increased right-to-left shunting of deoxygenated blood, decreased pulmonary blood flow, and increased systemic vascular resistance.

The typical triggers for cyanotic spells in infants and young children with TOF include:
- *Crying or agitation:* Increased sympathetic tone and increased oxygen demand can worsen right-to-left shunting and exacerbate cyanosis.
- *Feeding:* Increased oxygen demand during feeding can lead to decreased pulmonary blood flow and worsening cyanosis.
- *Exercise or exertion*: Physical activity can increase oxygen demand and worsen cyanosis.

Clinical manifestations of cyanotic spells may include:
- *Cyanosis:* Bluish discoloration of the skin, lips, and mucous membranes due to decreased oxygen saturation.
- *Respiratory distress:* Tachypnea (rapid breathing), dyspnea (shortness of breath), and respiratory distress may occur due to hypoxemia.
- *Irritability or agitation:* Infants may become fussy or irritable during cyanotic spells.
- *Syncope or loss of consciousness:* Severe hypoxemia can lead to loss of consciousness in some cases.

Management of cyanotic spells typically involves addressing the underlying cause (e.g., correcting dehydration and relieving airway obstruction) and providing supplemental oxygen to alleviate hypoxemia. In cases of severe cyanotic spells, interventions aimed at increasing systemic vascular resistance and reducing right-to-left shunting may be necessary. These interventions may include:
- *Knee-to-chest position:* Placing the child in a knee-to-chest position can increase systemic vascular resistance and improve pulmonary blood flow.
- *Oxygen therapy:* Administration of supplemental oxygen can alleviate hypoxemia and improve oxygen delivery to tissues.
- *IV fluids:* Administering IV fluids can help correct dehydration and increase intravascular volume, which may improve cardiac output and systemic perfusion.
- *Sedation*: Administering sedatives or analgesics may help calm the child and reduce agitation, thereby decreasing oxygen demand.

In severe cases refractory to medical management, emergency interventions such as IV morphine administration or even emergent surgical interventions to relieve obstruction (e.g., balloon valvuloplasty for pulmonary stenosis) may be necessary to stabilize the child and prevent further deterioration.

Overall, cyanotic spells are critical events in infants and children with congenital heart defects, particularly TOF, and require prompt recognition and appropriate management to prevent complications and optimize outcomes. Close monitoring and follow-up with a pediatric cardiologist are essential for infants and children with TOF to detect and manage cyanotic spells effectively.

Q 2. Endothelial receptor antagonists. *(Refer 2010/2019 MUHS)*

Ans. Endothelial receptor antagonists are a class of medications that target receptors on the endothelial cells lining blood vessels. These receptors play crucial roles in regulating vascular tone, endothelial function, and cardiovascular homeostasis. By blocking these receptors, endothelial receptor antagonists exert various effects on the cardiovascular system, making them valuable therapeutic agents for several cardiovascular conditions. Two prominent types of endothelial receptor antagonists are—(1) endothelin receptor antagonists (ERAs) and (2) prostaglandin receptor antagonists.

Endothelin Receptor Antagonists
Endothelin is a potent vasoconstrictor peptide produced by endothelial cells, and dysregulation of the endothelin system is implicated in various cardiovascular diseases. ERAs selectively block endothelin receptors, primarily endothelin receptor type A (ETA) and type B (ETB), thereby inhibiting the vasoconstrictive and profibrotic effects of endothelin.

Examples of ERAs:
- Bosentan
- Ambrisentan
- Macitentan

Clinical uses:
- *Pulmonary arterial hypertension (PAH)*: ERAs are approved for the treatment of PAH, where they help dilate pulmonary arteries, reduce pulmonary vascular resistance, and improve exercise capacity and quality of life in affected individuals.
- *Digital ulcers in systemic sclerosis:* Bosentan is approved for the treatment of digital ulcers in patients with systemic sclerosis (scleroderma).

Adverse effects: Common adverse effects of ERAs include liver enzyme abnormalities, peripheral edema, headache, nasal congestion, and anemia.

Regular monitoring of liver function tests is essential during treatment with ERAs due to the risk of hepatotoxicity.

Prostacyclin Receptor Antagonists
Prostacyclin (PGI2) is a vasodilator and inhibitor of platelet aggregation produced by endothelial cells. PGI2 receptor antagonists block the effects of PGI2, leading to vasoconstriction and platelet activation.

Example of a PGI2 receptor antagonist: Selexipag

Clinical uses: Pulmonary arterial hypertension: Selexipag is approved for the treatment of PAH, where it acts as a PGI2 receptor agonist, promoting vasodilation, and inhibiting platelet aggregation.

Adverse effects: Adverse effects of selexipag include headache, jaw pain, diarrhea, nausea, vomiting, and flushing. Titration of the dose is necessary to minimize adverse effects, and regular monitoring of liver function tests is recommended.

Conclusion: Endothelial receptor antagonists, including ERAs and PGI2 receptor antagonists, play essential roles in the management of PAH and other cardiovascular conditions characterized by endothelial dysfunction. While these medications offer significant benefits, they also carry the risk of adverse effects, necessitating careful patient selection, monitoring, and dose adjustment to optimize therapeutic outcomes and minimize risks.

Q 3. Starling's law.
(Refer 2009/2019 MUHS, 2018 MGR, 2016 Safdarjung)

Ans. Starling's law, also known as the Frank-Starling mechanism, describes the relationship between cardiac preload and stroke volume (SV), stating that the force of contraction of the heart muscle (myocardium) is directly proportional to its initial length or stretch, within physiological limits. In simpler terms, it means that the more the heart muscle fibers are stretched (due to an increase in preload), the stronger the force of contraction and the greater the volume of blood ejected from the heart with each beat.

Key Points of Starling's Law
- *Preload*: Preload refers to the degree of stretch of the cardiac muscle fibers just before contraction, typically determined by the volume of blood returning to the heart (venous return). Preload is influenced by factors such as blood volume, venous tone, and ventricular compliance.
- *Stroke volume*: SV is the amount of blood ejected from the ventricle with each heartbeat. It is determined by preload, afterload (resistance to ejection of blood from the ventricle), and myocardial contractility.

- *Direct relationship:* According to Starling's Law, there is a direct relationship between preload and SV. As preload increases (e.g., due to increased venous return or filling pressure), the myocardial fibers are stretched more, leading to increased force of contraction and greater SV.
- *Optimal length:* While increased preload initially leads to increased SV, there is an optimal length beyond which further stretching of the myocardial fibers does not result in increased force of contraction. This is because excessive stretching can lead to sarcomere overstretching and impaired contractility (the length-tension relationship).
- *Physiological significance:* Starling's Law ensures that the heart is capable of adjusting its output to match the volume of blood returning to it, thereby maintaining cardiac output and systemic perfusion in response to changes in venous return.

Clinical Implications
- *Heart failure*: In heart failure, impaired contractility leads to decreased SV and cardiac output. Starling's law may be partially responsible for compensatory mechanisms that attempt to maintain cardiac output by increasing preload, such as fluid retention and neurohormonal activation.
- *Treatment*: Drugs that affect preload, such as diuretics and vasodilators, are commonly used in the management of heart failure to optimize preload and reduce cardiac workload. However, excessive preload reduction may compromise SV and cardiac output.
- *Intraoperative management*: During surgery, optimizing preload is essential for maintaining adequate cardiac output and tissue perfusion. Monitoring preload using parameters such as central venous pressure (CVP) or pulmonary artery wedge pressure (PAWP) helps guide fluid management strategies.

In summary, Starling's Law describes the relationship between preload and SV, stating that an increase in preload leads to an increase in the force of contraction and SV up to a certain point. Understanding Starling's Law is crucial for managing conditions affecting cardiac function, such as heart failure, and optimizing fluid management in clinical settings.

Q 4. Athlete's heart. *(Refer 2010/2019 MUHS)*

Ans. Athlete's heart, also known as athletic heart syndrome, refers to a set of cardiovascular adaptations that occur in response to regular and vigorous physical training or athletic conditioning. These adaptations are generally considered physiological and are a normal response to exercise training rather than indicative of underlying cardiac pathology. Athlete's heart is characterized by specific changes in cardiac structure and function that enhance cardiovascular performance.

Key Features of Athlete's Heart
- *Cardiac hypertrophy:* One of the hallmark features of athlete's heart is cardiac hypertrophy, particularly of the left ventricle. This hypertrophy is typically concentric in nature, involving thickening of the left ventricular (LV) wall, and is primarily attributed to the hemodynamic effects of endurance training, including increased cardiac output and systemic arterial pressure.
- *Increased cardiac dimensions:* Athlete's heart may be associated with increased cardiac dimensions, including increased LV mass, cavity size, and wall thickness. These changes reflect the heart's adaptation to the increased demands of exercise and serve to optimize SV and cardiac output.
- *Bradycardia:* Athlete's heart is often accompanied by bradycardia, or a resting heart rate below the normal range for sedentary individuals. This is a result of increased vagal tone and enhanced parasympathetic activity, which occur in response to regular aerobic exercise training.
- *Normal or enhanced cardiac function*: Despite the structural changes observed in athlete's heart, cardiac function is typically normal or even enhanced. Athletes often exhibit increased LV ejection fraction, improved diastolic function, and enhanced cardiac reserve, allowing for greater exercise capacity and performance.
- *Electrocardiographic (ECG) changes:* ECG changes are common in athlete's heart and may include sinus bradycardia, increased vagal tone (e.g., prominent vagal maneuvers such as sinus arrhythmia or sinus arrest), and various repolarization abnormalities such as increased amplitude of R waves, increased voltage, and T-wave inversion, particularly in leads V1–V4.

Distinguishing Athlete's Heart from Pathological Conditions
While athlete's heart represents physiological adaptations to exercise training, it is important to distinguish it from pathological conditions that may mimic its features, such as hypertrophic cardiomyopathy (HCM) or dilated cardiomyopathy (DCM). Key differences include:
- *Symptoms*: Athlete's heart is typically asymptomatic and is not associated with adverse cardiovascular events, whereas patients with HCM or DCM may present with symptoms such as dyspnea, chest pain, palpitations, or syncope.
- *Family history:* Athlete's heart is not typically associated with a family history of sudden cardiac death or inherited cardiac conditions, whereas HCM and DCM often have a strong genetic component.
- *Diagnostic testing:* Differential diagnosis may require additional testing such as echocardiography, cardiac magnetic resonance imaging (MRI),

or genetic testing to differentiate between athlete's heart and pathological conditions.

Management

Management of athlete's heart involves regular monitoring to ensure that physiological adaptations do not progress to pathological conditions. This may include periodic clinical evaluation, ECG screening, and echocardiographic assessment to detect any abnormalities or changes over time. Education of athletes, coaches, and healthcare providers about the characteristics of athlete's heart and the importance of distinguishing it from pathological conditions is also essential.

In summary, athlete's heart represents a set of physiological adaptations to regular and vigorous exercise training, characterized by cardiac hypertrophy, increased cardiac dimensions, bradycardia, and normal or enhanced cardiac function. While these adaptations enhance cardiovascular performance, it is crucial to distinguish athlete's heart from pathological conditions to ensure appropriate management and minimize the risk of adverse cardiovascular events.

Q 5. Left ventricular remodeling. *(Refer 2019 MUHS, 2011/2013 MGR)*

Ans. LV remodeling refers to structural and functional changes that occur in the left ventricle of the heart in response to various pathological stimuli, such as myocardial infarction, hypertension, or chronic volume or pressure overload. LV remodeling involves alterations in ventricular size, shape, and function and is a key process in the progression of heart failure and other cardiovascular diseases.

Key Features of LV Remodeling
- *Ventricular dilatation*: LV remodeling often involves an increase in ventricular volume or dilatation, resulting from myocyte elongation, thinning of the ventricular wall, and enlargement of the ventricular cavity. Ventricular dilatation is typically associated with conditions such as myocardial infarction, where loss of myocardium leads to compensatory ventricular enlargement.
- *Hypertrophy*: LV remodeling may also involve hypertrophic changes, characterized by thickening of the ventricular wall and increased myocardial mass. Hypertrophy can be concentric, involving uniform thickening of the ventricular wall, or eccentric, characterized by asymmetric hypertrophy and ventricular dilatation. Hypertrophic remodeling is often seen in response to chronic pressure overload, such as in hypertension or aortic stenosis.
- *Changes in ventricular geometry*: LV remodeling can alter ventricular geometry, resulting in changes in ventricular shape and wall thickness.

These changes may affect ventricular function and contribute to the progression of heart failure. remodeling may result in abnormalities such as ventricular aneurysms, dyskinesia, or akinesia, which can further compromise cardiac function.
- *Altered ventricular function*: LV remodeling is associated with changes in ventricular systolic and diastolic function, which can impair cardiac performance and lead to symptoms of heart failure. These changes may include reduced ejection fraction, impaired contractility, increased ventricular stiffness, and diastolic dysfunction.
- *Neurohormonal activation*: LV remodeling is often accompanied by neurohormonal activation, including activation of the renin-angiotensin-aldosterone system (RAAS) and sympathetic nervous system. These neurohormonal changes contribute to myocardial fibrosis, inflammation, and oxidative stress, further exacerbating LV dysfunction and remodeling.

Clinical Implications
- *Heart failure*: LV remodeling is a central pathophysiological process in the development and progression of heart failure. Structural and functional changes associated with remodeling contribute to decreased cardiac output, increased ventricular filling pressures, and symptoms of heart failure.
- *Arrhythmias*: LV remodeling can predispose individuals to cardiac arrhythmias, including ventricular tachycardia and fibrillation, due to alterations in ventricular geometry, electrical instability, and conduction abnormalities.
- *Prognosis*: LV remodeling is associated with increased morbidity and mortality in patients with cardiovascular diseases. Assessment of LV remodeling, including ventricular size, function, and geometry, is important for risk stratification and guiding management strategies in these patients.

Management
- *Pharmacological therapy*: Pharmacological agents such as angiotensin-converting enzyme (ACE) inhibitors, angiotensin II receptor blockers (ARBs), beta-blockers, and mineralocorticoid receptor antagonists (MRAs) are commonly used to inhibit LV remodeling and improve outcomes in patients with heart failure and other cardiovascular diseases.
- *Device therapy*: In certain cases, device-based therapies such as cardiac resynchronization therapy (CRT) or implantable cardioverter-defibrillators (ICDs) may be indicated to optimize ventricular function, prevent arrhythmias, and reduce mortality in patients with LV remodeling and heart failure.

- *Surgical interventions*: Surgical interventions such as coronary artery bypass grafting (CABG), valve repair or replacement, and ventricular reconstruction surgery may be considered to address underlying causes of LV remodeling and improve cardiac function in selected patients.
- *Lifestyle modifications*: Lifestyle interventions such as regular exercise, dietary modifications (e.g., sodium restriction), smoking cessation, and weight management may help mitigate risk factors contributing to LV remodeling and improve overall cardiovascular health.

In summary, LV remodeling is a complex process involving structural and functional changes in the left ventricle in response to pathological stimuli. Understanding the mechanisms and clinical implications of LV remodeling is crucial for the management of heart failure and other cardiovascular diseases, with interventions aimed at preventing or reversing adverse remodeling and improving patient outcomes.

Q 6. Ankle brachial index. *(Refer 2011/2019 MUHS, 2013 Safdarjung)*

Ans. The ankle-brachial index (ABI) is a noninvasive diagnostic test used to assess peripheral arterial disease (PAD), which is a condition characterized by narrowing or blockage of the arteries supplying blood to the limbs, usually the legs. The ABI compares blood pressure measurements taken at the ankle and the brachial artery (in the arm) to evaluate the presence and severity of peripheral artery disease.

Procedure
- *Preparation:* The patient should lie down in a supine position for at least 5 minutes to allow for relaxation and stabilization of blood pressure.
- *Blood pressure measurement:* A blood pressure cuff is placed around the upper arm (brachial artery level) and around the ankles (dorsalis pedis and posterior tibial arteries). Doppler ultrasound is often used to detect the arterial pulses in the ankle arteries if they are not palpable.
- *Calculation of ABI*: The systolic blood pressure is recorded at the brachial artery and at each ankle artery. The ABI is calculated separately for each leg by dividing the highest systolic pressure at the ankle by the highest systolic pressure in the arm.

    ABI = Highest brachial systolic pressure/Highest ankle systolic pressure

- *Interpretation:*
    - *Normal ABI* typically ranges from 0.90 to 1.30.
    - *ABI <0.90* indicates PAD, with the severity increasing with lower values.
    - *ABI >1.30* may indicate non compressible arteries, often seen in patients with diabetes or medial arterial calcification.

Clinical Significance

- *Peripheral arterial disease diagnosis:* ABI is a sensitive and specific diagnostic tool for PAD. A lower ABI indicates reduced blood flow to the legs, suggesting the presence of PAD.
- *Assessment of disease severity:* The severity of PAD can be determined by the degree of reduction in ABI. Lower ABI values are associated with more severe PAD and an increased risk of adverse cardiovascular events, such as heart attack or stroke.
- *Risk stratification:* ABI is a useful tool for risk stratification in patients with PAD. Individuals with lower ABI values are at higher risk of complications, including limb ischemia, nonhealing wounds, and lower extremity amputation.
- *Monitoring response to treatment:* ABI can be used to monitor the response to treatment for PAD, such as lifestyle modifications, exercise therapy, medications, or revascularization procedures. Improvement in ABI values indicates successful treatment and improved blood flow to the legs.

In summary, the ABI is a simple, noninvasive test used to assess PAD by comparing blood pressure measurements in the ankle and arm. ABI is an essential tool for diagnosing PAD, assessing disease severity, risk stratification, and monitoring response to treatment in patients with peripheral artery disease.

SUGGESTED READING

1. Akazawa H, Komuro I. Navigational error in the heart leads to premature ventricular excitation. J Clin Investig. 2011;121(2):513-6.
2. Alver N, Bhagat R, Trager L, Brennan Z, Blitzer D, Louis C, et al. A primer for the student joining the congenital cardiac surgery service tomorrow: Primer 3 of 7. JTCVS Open. 2023;14:314-30.
3. Bloe CG. Use of pulmonary artery flotation catheters in the coronary care unit. Br J Nurs. 1994;3(16):810-5.
4. Brady W, Truwit JD, Brady W. Critical Decisions in Emergency and Acute Care Electrocardiography. United States: Wiley-Blackwell; 2009.
5. Capucci A. Clinical Cases in Cardiology. Philadelphia: Springer eBooks. Springer Nature; 2015.
6. Dokumen Pub. (2024). Pediatric Cardiology: Symptoms-Diagnosis-Treatment [1st ed]. [online] Available from https://dokumen.pub/pediatric-cardiology-symptoms-diagnosis-treatment-1stnbsped-9783131749512.html [Last accessed April, 2024].
7. Enabi J, Tahir M, Mukkera S, Garcia Fernandez A. A rare presentation of systemic sclerosis. Cureus. 2023;15(11):e48599.
8. Frank L, Dillman JR, Parish V, Mueller GC, Kazerooni EA, Bell A, et al. Cardiovascular MR imaging of conotruncal anomalies. Radiographics. 2010;30(4):1069-94.

9. Gatzoulis MA, Swan L, Therrien J, Pantely GA. Adult Congenital Heart Disease. New Jersey: Wiley eBooks; 2005.
10. Hsu PC, Lee WH, Lee HC, Tsai WC, Chu CY, Chen YC, et al. Association between modified CHA2DS2-VASc Score with Ankle-Brachial index < 0.9. Sci Rep. 2018;8(1):1175.
11. Liu C, Liu K, Ji Z, Liu G. Treatments for pulmonary arterial hypertension. Respiratory Medicine. 2006;100(5):765-74.
12. Moniuszko A, Kesala BA. Nuclear Cardiology Study Guide. Philadelphia: Springer Nature; 2014.
13. Singh SS, Pilkerton CS, Shrader CD, Frisbee SJ. Subclinical atherosclerosis, cardiovascular health, and disease risk: is there a case for the Cardiovascular Health Index in the primary prevention population? BMC Public Health. 2018;18(1).
14. Wiley Handbook of Current and Emerging Drug Therapies First published: 15 September 2006 Print ISBN: 9780470040980| Online ISBN: 9780470041000|DOI: 10.1002/9780470041000 Copyright © 2006 by John Wiley & Sons, Inc.

DM CARDIOLOGY EXAMINATION

Paper 1 (Set 2)

LONG-ESSAY QUESTIONS AND ANSWERS

Q 1. The development of the inter atrial septum, classify and describe the pathophysiology of various types of atrial septal defects.
(Refer 2020 MGR)

Ans. The development of the interatrial septum is a complex process that involves the formation and fusion of several embryonic structures. Understanding this developmental process is crucial for comprehending the various types of atrial septal defects (ASDs) and their associated pathophysiology.

Development of the Interatrial Septum
- *Primum and secundum septa:*
  - Initially, the heart starts as a simple tube. As it develops, the atria expand and become recognizable structures.
  - The primary septum, known as the septum primum, begins to form from the roof of the primitive atrium and grows downward toward the endocardial cushions.
  - Concurrently, another structure called the septum secundum forms to the right of the septum primum, partially overlapping it. This forms a one-way valve-like structure known as the foramen ovale, allowing blood to flow from the right atrium to the left atrium during fetal life.
- *Fusion and remodeling:*
  - As development progresses, the septum primum and septum secundum fuse together, closing the foramen ovale.
  - The remaining portion of the septum primum, called the valve of the foramen ovale, adheres to the septum secundum, ensuring a complete closure of the interatrial septum after birth.

Classification and Description of Atrial Septal Defects
- *Secundum ASD:*
  - This is the most common type of ASD and occurs due to incomplete fusion of the septum primum and septum secundum.
  - It leads to a direct communication between the right and left atria, usually through the fossa ovalis, resulting in a left-to-right shunt of blood.

- *Primum ASD:*
  - This defect occurs at the lower part of the atrial septum and is often associated with other congenital heart defects such as cleft mitral valve or endocardial cushion defects.
  - It is characterized by a defect in the AV septum, leading to a communication between the atria and ventricles.
- *Sinus venosus ASD:*
  - This type of ASD occurs near the junction of the superior vena cava and the right atrium or the inferior vena cava and the right atrium.
  - It is typically associated with anomalous pulmonary venous drainage.
- *Coronary sinus ASD:* This rare type of ASD involves an abnormal communication between the coronary sinus and the left atrium.

Pathophysiology of Atrial Septal Defects
- ASDs result in a left-to-right shunt of blood, allowing oxygenated blood from the left atrium to flow into the right atrium.
- This shunting of blood causes increased blood flow to the right side of the heart and pulmonary circulation, leading to volume overload of the right atrium and ventricle.
- Over time, if left untreated, ASDs can lead to complications such as pulmonary hypertension (PH), right-sided heart failure, atrial arrhythmias, and paradoxical embolism.

In summary, the development of the interatrial septum involves the fusion of various embryonic structures to form a complete partition between the right and left atria. Failure in this process leads to different types of ASDs, each with its own pathophysiology and clinical implications. Understanding these developmental and pathological aspects is essential for proper diagnosis and management of ASDs.

Q 2. Discuss the neurohumoral mechanisms operating in cardiac failure. *(Refer 2020 MGR)*

Ans. Cardiac failure, also known as heart failure, is a complex clinical syndrome characterized by the heart's inability to pump blood efficiently to meet the body's metabolic demands. Several neurohumoral mechanisms come into play in response to cardiac failure, attempting to compensate for the reduced cardiac output and maintain adequate tissue perfusion. However, these mechanisms, while initially adaptive, can exacerbate heart failure over time if left unchecked. Here is an elaboration on the neurohumoral mechanisms operating in cardiac failure:
- *Sympathetic nervous system (SNS) activation:*
  - In response to reduced cardiac output and decreased tissue perfusion, the SNS is activated.

- This activation leads to increased release of catecholamines, primarily norepinephrine, from sympathetic nerve terminals and the adrenal medulla.
- Norepinephrine acts on β1-adrenergic receptors in the heart, leading to increased heart rate, myocardial contractility, and systemic vasoconstriction.
- These responses initially help maintain cardiac output and blood pressure but can contribute to myocardial hypertrophy, increased oxygen demand, and worsening heart failure over time.
- *Renin-angiotensin-aldosterone system (RAAS) activation:*
  - Reduced renal perfusion and activation of the SNS stimulate the release of renin from the kidneys.
  - Renin acts on angiotensinogen to form angiotensin I, which is then converted to angiotensin II by ACE, primarily in the lungs.
  - Angiotensin II is a potent vasoconstrictor and stimulates the release of aldosterone from the adrenal cortex, leading to sodium and water retention in the kidneys.
  - These actions result in increased systemic vascular resistance, blood volume expansion, and preload on the heart, further exacerbating heart failure and contributing to fluid retention and edema.
- *Natriuretic peptides release:*
  - In response to increased atrial and ventricular wall tension, the heart releases atrial natriuretic peptide (ANP) and brain natriuretic peptide (BNP).
  - ANP and BNP act as counter-regulatory hormones to the RAAS and SNS, promoting vasodilation, natriuresis (excretion of sodium in the urine), and diuresis (increased urine output).
  - These effects help reduce preload and afterload on the heart, counteracting the compensatory mechanisms that contribute to heart failure progression.
  - However, in advanced heart failure, the compensatory release of ANP and BNP may become inadequate to offset the detrimental effects of SNS activation and RAAS overactivity.
- *Endothelin release:*
  - Endothelin is a potent vasoconstrictor released by endothelial cells in response to various stimuli, including inflammation, hypoxia, and shear stress.
  - In heart failure, endothelin levels are often elevated, contributing to vasoconstriction, increased systemic vascular resistance, and impaired endothelial function.
  - Endothelin antagonists are used in the treatment of heart failure to counteract these effects and improve hemodynamic parameters.

Overall, the neurohumoral mechanisms operating in cardiac failure involve a complex interplay between the SNS, RAAS, natriuretic peptides, and endothelin. While initially adaptive, these mechanisms can contribute to the progression of heart failure if left unchecked. Targeted pharmacological interventions aim to modulate these pathways to improve cardiac function and outcomes in patients with heart failure.

SHORT QUESTIONS AND ANSWERS

Q 1. Cardiac conduction system and blood supply. *(Refer 2020 MGR)*

Ans. The cardiac conduction system is a specialized network of cells responsible for generating and coordinating the electrical impulses that regulate the heartbeat. This system ensures that the heart contracts rhythmically and efficiently, allowing for effective blood pumping throughout the body. The key components of the cardiac conduction system include the sinoatrial (SA) node, atrioventricular (AV) node, bundle of His, bundle branches, and Purkinje fibers.

- *SA node*:
  - Located in the right atrium near the opening of the superior vena cava.
  - Serves as the heart's natural pacemaker, initiating electrical impulses that travel through the atria, causing them to contract and pump blood into the ventricles.
- *AV node*:
  - Located at the junction of the atria and ventricles
  - It acts as a gateway, delaying the transmission of electrical impulses to the ventricles, allowing time for the atria to fully contract before ventricular contraction begins.
  - *Bundle of His*: A bundle of specialized fibers that transmit the electrical impulses from the AV node to the ventricles.
  - *Bundle branches*: Divisions of the bundle of His that conduct electrical impulses to the left and right ventricles.
  - *Purkinje fibers*: Specialized cardiac muscle fibers that rapidly transmit electrical impulses throughout the ventricles, causing coordinated ventricular contraction.

Blood supply to the cardiac conduction system is crucial for its proper function and viability. The conduction system receives its blood supply from the coronary arteries, which originate from the aorta and supply oxygenated blood to the heart muscle. Specifically:

- The SA node is predominantly supplied by the right coronary artery (in about 60–70% of individuals) or the left circumflex artery.

- The AV node receives blood primarily from the right coronary artery in most individuals.
- The bundle of His, bundle branches, and Purkinje fibers are supplied by branches of the left and right coronary arteries, ensuring adequate oxygenation for proper conduction function.

Impairment of blood flow to the cardiac conduction system, such as in coronary artery disease, can lead to conduction abnormalities, arrhythmias, and even complete heart block. Thus, maintaining healthy coronary circulation is essential for the proper functioning of the cardiac conduction system and overall cardiac health.

Q 2. Culture negative endocarditis. *(Refer 2019 MGR)*

Ans. Culture-negative endocarditis (CNE) refers to a clinical condition where infective endocarditis is suspected based on clinical signs and symptoms, but routine blood cultures fail to identify the causative microorganism. Despite advances in diagnostic techniques, approximately 5–31% of cases of infective endocarditis remain culture negative.

Causes and contributing factors:
- *Prior antibiotic use:* Patients may have received antibiotics before blood cultures are drawn, inhibiting microbial growth.
- *Fastidious organisms*: Some pathogens have specific growth requirements and may not grow in standard blood culture media.
- *Noninfectious causes:* CNE may result from noninfectious conditions such as Libman-Sacks endocarditis (associated with systemic lupus erythematosus), marantic endocarditis (associated with hypercoagulable states), or cardiac tumors.
- *Microbial characteristics:* Some microorganisms, such as *Bartonella* species or *Coxiella burnetii*, have prolonged incubation periods and may require specialized culture techniques for detection.

Diagnostic approach:
- *Clinical evaluation:* Careful clinical assessment, including history, physical examination, and echocardiography, is essential for diagnosing endocarditis.
- *Serological tests:* Serological assays, including antibody detection and polymerase chain reaction (PCR) assays, can aid in the diagnosis of specific pathogens such as *Bartonella* or *Coxiella burnetii*.
- *Imaging studies:* Echocardiography, including transthoracic echocardiography (TTE) and transesophageal echocardiography (TEE), is critical for detecting valvular vegetations and other cardiac abnormalities associated with endocarditis.

- *Empirical therapy:* Empirical antibiotic therapy targeting common pathogens associated with endocarditis may be initiated based on clinical suspicion, pending further diagnostic evaluation.

Management:
- *Antibiotic therapy:* Treatment should be guided by clinical suspicion, epidemiological factors, and available microbiological data, if any. Empirical antibiotic therapy is often initiated pending further diagnostic evaluation.
- *Surgical intervention:* Surgical management, including valve repair or replacement, may be necessary in cases of severe valvular dysfunction, heart failure, or complications such as abscess formation or persistent infection.
- *Close follow-up:* Patients with CNE require close monitoring to assess treatment response, evaluate for complications, and guide further management decisions.

In summary, CNE poses diagnostic and therapeutic challenges. A systematic approach, including clinical evaluation, advanced imaging techniques, serological assays, and empirical antibiotic therapy, is essential for accurate diagnosis and effective management of this condition. Collaboration between infectious disease specialists, cardiologists, and other healthcare providers is crucial to optimize patient outcomes.

Q 3. Koch's triangle. *(Refer 2020 MGR, 2016/2017/2019 Safdarjung)*

Ans. Koch's triangle is a structural region of the heart located in the right atrium and is important in the anatomical arrangement of the cardiac conduction system. It is named after the German physician Walter Karl Koch who described it in 1910. Koch's triangle serves as a landmark for the location of the AV node, one of the key components of the cardiac conduction system responsible for electrical impulse propagation from the atria to the ventricles.

Anatomy of Koch's triangle:
- *Superior border:* The superior border of Koch's triangle is formed by the tendon of Todaro, which is a fibrous band extending from the central fibrous body to the anterior rim of the oval fossa (also known as the fossa ovalis).
- *Inferior border:* The inferior border is formed by the coronary sinus orifice, where the coronary sinus, a large venous structure draining blood from the heart muscle, enters the right atrium.
- *Septal border:* The septal border of Koch's triangle is formed by the septal cusp of the tricuspid valve, which is one of the three leaflets of the tricuspid valve separating the right atrium from the right ventricle.

Significance:
- *Location of the AV node:* Koch's triangle serves as a landmark for the location of the AV node, which is situated at the apex of the triangle, near the ostium of the coronary sinus. This anatomical arrangement facilitates the efficient transmission of electrical impulses from the atria to the ventricles.
- *Clinical relevance:* Koch's triangle is clinically relevant in electrophysiology procedures, such as catheter ablation for supraventricular tachycardias. The AV node's proximity to the triangle's apex makes it accessible for diagnostic and therapeutic interventions aimed at managing arrhythmias originating from this region.

In summary, Koch's triangle is an anatomical landmark in the right atrium of the heart, delineated by the tendon of Todaro, coronary sinus orifice, and septal cusp of the tricuspid valve. It plays a crucial role in defining the location of the AV node and is of clinical importance in electrophysiological procedures targeting arrhythmias involving the cardiac conduction system.

Q 4. Pulmonary vascular resistance. *(Refer 2009/2020 - MGR)*

Ans. Pulmonary vascular resistance (PVR) refers to the resistance exerted by the blood vessels in the pulmonary circulation. It is a critical parameter that influences pulmonary blood flow and pressures within the pulmonary vasculature. PVR is determined primarily by the diameter of the pulmonary arterioles, the viscosity of blood, and the length and compliance of the pulmonary vessels.

Factors influencing PVR:
- *Pulmonary arteriolar tone:* The primary determinant of PVR is the degree of constriction or dilation of the pulmonary arterioles. Constriction of these vessels increases resistance, whereas dilation decreases resistance. Factors such as hypoxia, acidosis, and PH can lead to increased pulmonary arteriolar tone and elevated PVR.
- *Blood viscosity:* Changes in blood viscosity, such as alterations in hematocrit or the presence of abnormal blood constituents, can impact PVR. Increased viscosity generally leads to increased resistance.
- *Vessel length and compliance:* The length and compliance (elasticity) of the pulmonary vessels also influence PVR. Longer vessels and decreased vessel compliance can contribute to elevated resistance.

Clinical significance:
- *Pulmonary hypertension*: Elevated PVR is a hallmark feature of PH, a condition characterized by increased pressure in the pulmonary arteries.

High PVR contributes to right ventricular strain and can lead to right-sided heart failure if left untreated.
- *Congenital heart disease:* In certain congenital heart defects, such as VSD or patent ductus arteriosus, elevated PVR can impede normal blood flow patterns and contribute to pulmonary overcirculation. Conversely, conditions such as pulmonary atresia or pulmonary stenosis can result in increased PVR and reduced pulmonary blood flow.
- *Respiratory disorders:* Respiratory conditions such as acute respiratory distress syndrome (ARDS) or chronic obstructive pulmonary disease (COPD) can lead to changes in PVR due to alterations in lung mechanics, gas exchange, and pulmonary vascular tone.

Measurement of PVR

Pulmonary vascular resistance is typically assessed using invasive hemodynamic monitoring techniques, such as right heart catheterization. It is calculated using the following formula:

$$PVR = \frac{\text{Mean pulmonary arterial pressure (mPAP)} - \text{pulmonary capillary wedge pressure (PCWP)}}{\text{Cardiac output (CO)}}$$

where mPAP is the mean pulmonary arterial pressure, PCWP is the pulmonary capillary wedge pressure, and CO is the cardiac output.

In summary, PVR is a critical determinant of pulmonary blood flow and pressures. Understanding PVR and its regulation is essential for the diagnosis and management of various cardiopulmonary conditions, particularly PH.

Q 5. Pathology of vulnerable plaque.   *(Refer 2015/2020 - MGR)*

Ans. Vulnerable plaques are a subtype of atherosclerotic plaques that are particularly prone to rupture, leading to acute cardiovascular events such as myocardial infarction or stroke. Understanding the pathology of vulnerable plaques is crucial for identifying individuals at high risk of these life-threatening events and developing strategies for prevention and treatment.

Pathological features of vulnerable plaques:
- *Thin fibrous cap*: Vulnerable plaques typically have a thin fibrous cap covering a lipid-rich necrotic core. The fibrous cap is composed of smooth muscle cells, collagen, and elastin. A thin fibrous cap is prone to rupture due to mechanical stress and inflammation.
- *Inflammation*: Vulnerable plaques are characterized by a high degree of inflammation within the plaque and surrounding tissue. Inflammatory cells, such as macrophages and T lymphocytes, infiltrate the plaque and release cytokines and enzymes that weaken the fibrous cap and promote plaque instability.

- *Lipid-rich core:* The core of vulnerable plaques contains a large amount of lipid-laden macrophages, cholesterol crystals, and extracellular lipid deposits. These lipid-rich regions are prone to rupture and thrombus formation, leading to occlusion of the coronary artery or cerebral vessel.
- *Neovascularization:* Vulnerable plaques often exhibit neovascularization, the formation of new blood vessels within the plaque. These fragile vessels are leaky and prone to hemorrhage, contributing to plaque destabilization and thrombosis.
- *Plaque erosion versus plaque rupture:* Vulnerable plaques can lead to acute cardiovascular events through two main mechanisms—plaque erosion and plaque rupture. Plaque erosion occurs when the endothelial lining of the artery is disrupted, exposing the underlying plaque to the bloodstream, leading to platelet aggregation and thrombus formation. Plaque rupture involves the rupture of the fibrous cap, exposing the lipid-rich core to the bloodstream, resulting in platelet activation, thrombosis, and vessel occlusion.

Clinical implications:
- *Acute coronary syndromes*: Vulnerable plaques are a major underlying cause of acute coronary syndromes, such as unstable angina, myocardial infarction, and sudden cardiac death.
- *Ischemic stroke*: Vulnerable plaques in the carotid or cerebral arteries can rupture, leading to embolic stroke or thrombotic occlusion of the vessel.
- *Risk stratification*: Identifying individuals with vulnerable plaques is crucial for risk stratification and implementing preventive measures, such as lifestyle modifications, statin therapy, antiplatelet agents, and revascularization procedures.

In summary, vulnerable plaques are characterized by specific pathological features, including a thin fibrous cap, inflammation, lipid-rich core, neovascularization, and propensity for rupture. Understanding the pathology of vulnerable plaques is essential for identifying high-risk individuals and implementing strategies to prevent acute cardiovascular events.

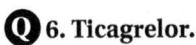 **6. Ticagrelor.** *(Refer 2020 MGR)*

Ans. Ticagrelor is a medication used in the management of acute coronary syndromes, particularly in patients with unstable angina or myocardial infarction (heart attack), and those undergoing percutaneous coronary intervention (PCI) with stent placement. It belongs to the class of medications known as antiplatelet drugs, specifically the P2Y12 receptor inhibitors.

Mechanism of action: Ticagrelor exerts its therapeutic effects by irreversibly binding to the P2Y12 receptors on platelets, thereby inhibiting adenosine diphosphate (ADP)-mediated platelet activation and aggregation. This inhibition reduces the risk of thrombus formation, which is crucial in preventing further occlusion of coronary arteries and subsequent cardiovascular events.

Pharmacokinetics:
- Ticagrelor is administered orally and is rapidly absorbed after ingestion.
- It has a bioavailability of approximately 36%, with peak plasma concentrations achieved within 1–2 hours after dosing.
- Ticagrelor is extensively metabolized in the liver via cytochrome P450 enzymes, primarily CYP3A4 and CYP3A5, to its active metabolite.
- The active metabolite contributes significantly to ticagrelor's antiplatelet effects.
- Ticagrelor and its active metabolite have elimination half-lives of approximately 7–8 hours and 9 hours, respectively.

Clinical uses:
- Ticagrelor is indicated for the prevention of thrombotic cardiovascular events in patients with acute coronary syndromes (unstable angina, non-ST-segment elevation myocardial infarction, and ST-segment elevation myocardial infarction), including those managed medically or undergoing PCI.
- It is often prescribed in combination with aspirin as dual antiplatelet therapy to reduce the risk of recurrent cardiovascular events.

Adverse effects:
- Common adverse effects of ticagrelor include bleeding, dyspnea, bradycardia, and transient increases in serum uric acid levels.
- Ticagrelor may also cause ventricular pauses and asymptomatic ventricular pauses on electrocardiogram monitoring, which typically resolve spontaneously.
- There is a small increased risk of intracranial bleeding with ticagrelor compared to other P2Y12 inhibitors.

Contraindications:
- Ticagrelor is contraindicated in patients with a history of intracranial bleeding and active pathological bleeding.
- It should be used with caution in patients with a history of asthma or COPD due to the risk of dyspnea.

In summary, ticagrelor is an antiplatelet medication used in the management of acute coronary syndromes to reduce the risk of thrombotic cardiovascular events. It exerts its effects by inhibiting platelet aggregation through irreversible binding to P2Y12 receptors. Ticagrelor is generally well-tolerated but may cause bleeding and dyspnea as adverse effects.

Q 7. Aortitis. *(Refer 2011/2020 MGR)*

Ans. Aortitis refers to inflammation of the aorta, the largest artery in the body. It can result from various underlying causes, including infectious, autoimmune, and idiopathic conditions, and can affect any segment of the aorta, including the ascending aorta, aortic arch, descending thoracic aorta, and abdominal aorta.

Causes:
- *Infectious aortitis*: Caused by bacterial, viral, fungal, or parasitic infections. Common pathogens include *Treponema pallidum* (syphilis), *Salmonella* species, *Mycobacterium tuberculosis*, and certain viruses.
- *Autoimmune aortitis:* Associated with autoimmune diseases such as giant cell arteritis, Takayasu arteritis, and rheumatoid arthritis.
- *Idiopathic aortitis*: Inflammation of the aorta with no identifiable cause. It may represent a localized form of vasculitis or be related to other systemic inflammatory conditions.

Clinical presentation:
- Aortitis may present with nonspecific symptoms such as fever, fatigue, malaise, weight loss, and generalized inflammatory symptoms.
- Symptoms can vary depending on the location and severity of aortic involvement. Complications may include aortic aneurysm, aortic dissection, or rupture.

Diagnosis:
- Diagnosis of aortitis typically involves a combination of clinical evaluation, imaging studies, laboratory tests, and sometimes histopathological examination.
- Imaging modalities such as computed tomography (CT), MRI, or positron emission tomography (PET) may demonstrate thickening of the aortic wall, aneurysmal changes, or signs of inflammation.
- Laboratory tests may show elevated inflammatory markers such as erythrocyte sedimentation rate (ESR) and C-reactive protein (CRP).
- Definitive diagnosis often requires biopsy of the affected tissue, but this is not always feasible or necessary.

Treatment:
- Treatment of aortitis depends on the underlying cause and severity of inflammation.
- Infectious aortitis typically requires antimicrobial therapy targeting the causative pathogen.
- Autoimmune aortitis may require immunosuppressive therapy with corticosteroids or other immunomodulatory agents.

- Management of idiopathic aortitis focuses on controlling inflammation and preventing complications such as aortic aneurysm or dissection. This may involve anti-inflammatory medications and regular monitoring with imaging studies.

In summary, aortitis is a condition characterized by inflammation of the aorta, with diverse etiologies and clinical presentations. Prompt diagnosis and appropriate management are essential to prevent complications and preserve aortic integrity.

Q 8. Electrocardiographic criteria of right ventricular hypertrophy.
(Refer 2020 - MGR)

Ans. Electrocardiographic criteria for diagnosing right ventricular hypertrophy (RVH) involve assessing specific changes in the electrical activity of the heart indicative of increased muscle mass or workload in the right ventricle. RVH may result from various conditions such as PH, congenital heart disease, or chronic lung diseases.

Key ECG criteria for RVH:
- *Increased R-wave amplitude in leads V1 or V2:* Normally, lead V1 typically shows a predominantly negative deflection (S wave) due to the rightward orientation of the heart. In RVH, there is often a prominent R wave, leading to a tall R wave in V1 (>7 mm).
- *Deep S-wave in lead V6:* Lead V6 typically shows a predominant R wave due to the leftward orientation of the heart. In RVH, there may be a deep S wave in lead V6 (>2.5 mm), reflecting increased electrical forces directed away from the left ventricle.
- *Right axis deviation:* A deviation of the QRS axis to the right (>+110 degrees) indicates increased electrical activity in the right ventricle.
- *P-pulmonale*: P-pulmonale refers to the presence of peaked or tall P waves in the inferior leads (II, III, and aVF), suggestive of right atrial enlargement secondary to increased right ventricular pressure.
- *Incomplete or complete right bundle branch block (RBBB):* RBBB may be present due to delayed conduction through the hypertrophied right ventricle.
- *T-wave changes*: T-wave inversion in leads V1–V4 may occur in advanced cases of RVH.

Note: While these criteria may suggest the presence of RVH, they are not specific and may be influenced by factors such as age, gender, and body habitus. Confirmation of RVH typically requires additional imaging studies such as echocardiography or cardiac MRI.

In summary, ECG criteria for RVH involve specific changes in the electrical patterns observed on the electrocardiogram, including increased R-wave amplitude in leads V1 or V2, deep S-wave in lead V6, right axis deviation, P-pulmonale, incomplete or complete RBBB, and T-wave changes. These criteria, when interpreted in conjunction with clinical findings and imaging studies, aid in the diagnosis and management of RVH.

Q 9. Hypocalcemia. *(Refer 2020 - MGR)*

Ans. Hypocalcemia refers to a condition characterized by low levels of calcium in the blood. Calcium is an essential mineral involved in various physiological processes, including bone health, muscle function, nerve transmission, and blood clotting. Hypocalcemia can result from various underlying causes and may manifest with a range of symptoms and complications.

Causes:
- *Hypoparathyroidism*: Reduced production or secretion of parathyroid hormone (PTH), which regulates calcium levels in the blood.
- *Vitamin D deficiency*: Inadequate intake or absorption of vitamin D, which is necessary for calcium absorption from the intestines.
- *Chronic kidney disease*: Impaired kidney function can lead to decreased activation of vitamin D and reduced renal calcium excretion.
- *Acute pancreatitis*: Calcium can bind to fatty acids released during pancreatitis, leading to precipitation and hypocalcemia.
- *Hypomagnesemia*: Magnesium deficiency can impair PTH secretion and action, leading to hypocalcemia.
- *Alkalosis*: Respiratory or metabolic alkalosis can cause a shift of ionized calcium into cells, reducing serum calcium levels.
- *Medications*: Certain medications, such as loop diuretics, bisphosphonates, and antiepileptic drugs, can affect calcium metabolism and lead to hypocalcemia.

Clinical manifestations:
- *Neuromuscular symptoms*: Tetany, muscle cramps, paresthesias, and positive Chvostek's and Trousseau's signs due to increased neuromuscular excitability
- *Cardiovascular symptoms*: Prolonged QT interval, arrhythmias (e.g., ventricular tachycardia), and heart failure in severe cases
- *Neurological symptoms*: Seizures, confusion, irritability, and depression
- *Dermatological manifestations*: Dry skin, coarse hair, and brittle nails
- *Cataracts*: Chronic hypocalcemia may lead to the development of cataracts.

Diagnosis:
- Serum calcium levels below the normal range (usually <8.5 mg/dL or <2.125 mmol/L) confirm the diagnosis of hypocalcemia.
- Measurement of ionized calcium levels provides a more accurate assessment of calcium status.
- Evaluation of magnesium levels and other electrolytes may help identify underlying causes.

Treatment:
- Treatment of hypocalcemia aims to correct the underlying cause and replenish calcium levels.
- Oral or IV calcium supplementation may be administered depending on the severity of symptoms and underlying etiology.
- Vitamin D supplementation is often necessary, particularly in cases of vitamin D deficiency.
- Management of associated electrolyte imbalances, such as hypomagnesemia, is essential.

In summary, hypocalcemia is characterized by low levels of calcium in the blood and can result from various underlying causes. Prompt recognition and appropriate management are crucial to prevent complications and alleviate symptoms associated with hypocalcemia.

Q 10. Anatomy of the left ventricle. *(Refer 2020 MGR)*

Ans. The left ventricle is one of the four chambers of the heart responsible for pumping oxygenated blood to the rest of the body. It is located in the lower left portion of the heart and plays a vital role in maintaining systemic circulation. The anatomy of the left ventricle is specialized to accommodate the high pressures generated during systole while ensuring efficient blood ejection.

Anatomical features:
- *Shape and size:* The left ventricle has a conical shape, with its apex directed inferiorly and anteriorly toward the left side of the chest. It is larger and thicker-walled than the right ventricle due to the higher pressures required to pump blood throughout the systemic circulation.
- *Wall thickness:* The muscular wall of the left ventricle is much thicker than that of the right ventricle, reflecting its role in generating the high pressures necessary to propel blood through the systemic circulation. The LV wall is composed of three layers—(1) the endocardium (inner layer), (2) myocardium (middle layer), and (3) epicardium (outer layer).
- *Chamber dimensions:* The LV cavity is elliptical in shape when viewed from the front (anterior) aspect and circular when viewed from the side (lateral) aspect. It typically measures around 4-6 cm in diameter and 1-1.5 cm in thickness in adults.

- *Valves and papillary muscles*: The left ventricle contains the mitral valve, which separates it from the left atrium and regulates blood flow during diastole. The mitral valve consists of two cusps (anterior and posterior) anchored to the papillary muscles by chordae tendineae. The papillary muscles prevent the mitral valve from prolapsing into the left atrium during ventricular contraction.
- *Blood supply:* The left ventricle receives oxygenated blood from the left atrium via the mitral valve and pumps it into the aorta through the aortic valve. The coronary arteries, including the left anterior descending artery and the circumflex artery, supply oxygen-rich blood to the myocardium of the left ventricle.

Function:
- During systole, the left ventricle contracts forcefully, generating high pressures to eject blood into the aorta and systemic circulation.
- The left ventricle relaxes during diastole, allowing blood to flow from the left atrium through the open mitral valve and fill the ventricular chamber in preparation for the next contraction.

In summary, the left ventricle is a vital component of the heart responsible for pumping oxygenated blood to the systemic circulation. Its specialized anatomy enables it to withstand high pressures and efficiently propel blood throughout the body, contributing to overall cardiovascular function.

SUGGESTED READING

1. ACC/AHA guidelines for the management of patients with valvular heart disease. A report of the American College of Cardiology/American Heart Association. Task Force on Practice Guidelines (Committee on Management of Patients with Valvular Heart Disease). J Am Coll Cardiol. 1998;32(5):1486-582.
2. Al-Naamani K, Hijal T, Nguyen V, Andrew S, Nguyen T, Huynh T. Predictive values of the electrocardiogram in diagnosing pulmonary hypertension. Int J Cardiol. 2008;127(2):214-8.
3. Brady WJ, Lipinski MJ, Darby AE, Bond MC, Charlton NP, Hudson K, et al. Electrocardiogram in Clinical Medicine. Philadelphia: Wiley; 2020.
4. Castellano JM, Kovacic JC, Sanz J, Fuster V. Are we ignoring the dilated thoracic aorta? Ann N Y Acad Sci. 2012;1254(1):164-74.
5. Manning-Tobin JJ, Moore KJ, Seimon TA, Bell SA, Sharuk M, Alvarez-Leite JI, et al. Loss of SR-A and CD36 Activity Reduces Atherosclerotic Lesion Complexity Without Abrogating Foam Cell Formation in Hyperlipidemic Mice. Arterioscler, Thromb, Vasc Biol. 2009;29(1):19-26.
6. Manning WJ. Role of Transesophageal Echocardiography in the Management of Thromboembolic Stroke. Am J Cardiol. 1997;80(4):19D-28D.
7. Mazur W, Siegel MJ, Miszalski-Jamka T, Pelberg R. CT Atlas of Adult Congenital Heart Disease. Philadelphia. Springer Nature; (2013).
8. Morady F. Fast pathway ablation for atrioventricular node reentrant tachycardia. J Am Coll Cardiol. 1995;25(5):982-3.

9. Oprea AD, Popescu WM. ADP-Receptor Inhibitors in the Perioperative Period: The Good, the Bad, and the Ugly. J Cardiothorac Vasc Anesth. 2013;27(4):779-95.
10. Sapna FNU, Raveena FNU, Chandio M, Bai K, Sayyar, M, Varrassi G, et al. Advancements in Heart Failure Management: A Comprehensive Narrative Review of Emerging Therapies. Cureus. 2023;15(10):e46486.
11. Shu T, Zhou Y, Yan C. The perspective of cAMP/cGMP signaling and cyclic nucleotide phosphodiesterases in aortic aneurysm and dissection. Vasc Pharmacol. 2024;154:107278-8.
12. Silva C. (2020). Hypoparathyroidism Test Should be Given to Type 2 Diabetes Patients. [online] Available from https://hypoparathyroidismnews.com/news/type-2-diabetes-patients-should-have-calcium-test-for-hypoparathyroidism/ [Last accessed April, 2024].
13. Townend JN, Griffith MJ. The diagnosis of bradycardias and their management. Curr Anaesth Crit Care. 1995;6(3):148-54.
14. Wilber DJ, Kall JG, Cooke PA. Electroanatomic imaging using magnetic catheter tracking in the diagnosis and treatment of atrial arrhythmias. J Electrocardiol. 1998;31:92-100.

DM CARDIOLOGY EXAMINATION

Paper 1 (Set 3)

LONG-ESSAY QUESTIONS AND ANSWERS

Q 1. Discuss embryology, classification, pathophysiology and management of patent ductus arteriosus. *(Refer 2021-MUHS)*

Ans. Patent ductus arteriosus (PDA) is a congenital heart defect characterized by the persistence of the ductus arteriosus, a fetal blood vessel that normally connects the pulmonary artery to the descending aorta during fetal development. This connection allows for the bypass of the nonfunctional fetal lungs. However, in a normal course of development, the ductus arteriosus usually closes shortly after birth. When it remains open (patent), it can lead to significant physiological problems.

- *Embryology:* During fetal development, the ductus arteriosus is a crucial structure that allows for blood to bypass the nonfunctional lungs. In a typical scenario, the ductus arteriosus starts to close shortly after birth, usually within the first few days to weeks, facilitated by various physiological changes, such as increased oxygen levels. The closure is primarily mediated by constriction and then fibrosis of the vessel. Failure of this closure results in PDA.
- *Classification:* Patent ductus arteriosus can be classified based on various factors including:
  - *Size:* The size of the PDA can vary from small to large.
  - *Clinical presentation:* It can be asymptomatic or symptomatic.
  - *Associated conditions:* PDA can occur in isolation or be associated with other congenital heart defects or genetic syndromes.
- *Pathophysiology:* The persistence of the ductus arteriosus leads to abnormal blood flow between the aorta and the pulmonary artery. This causes an increase in pulmonary blood flow, leading to left-to-right shunting of blood. The left-to-right shunting can cause several complications including:
  - Volume overload of the left heart
  - Pulmonary hypertension
  - Risk of infective endocarditis
  - Risk of developing Eisenmenger syndrome if left untreated, which involves a reversal of the shunt leading to right-to-left flow and cyanosis.
- *Management:* Management of PDA depends on various factors including the size of the defect, the presence of symptoms, associated complications, and the overall health of the patient. Management options include:

- *Medical management:* In some cases, especially in premature infants or small PDAs, medical management may be attempted. This typically involves administering medications such as indomethacin or ibuprofen, which help promote closure of the ductus arteriosus by inhibiting prostaglandin synthesis.
- *Surgical closure:* Surgical closure is often recommended for larger PDAs, or those that do not respond to medical management. The procedure involves making an incision in the chest, locating the PDA, and then tying it off or sealing it with sutures.
- *Transcatheter closure:* In recent years, transcatheter closure has become a common approach for closing PDAs, particularly in older children and adults. This minimally invasive procedure involves inserting a catheter through a blood vessel, usually in the groin, and guiding it to the PDA. A closure device, such as a coil or occluder, is then deployed to seal the PDA.
- *Monitoring and follow-up:* Regardless of the management approach, patients with PDA require regular monitoring and follow-up to assess for any residual shunting, complications, or recurrence.

In summary, PDA is a congenital heart defect characterized by the persistence of the ductus arteriosus after birth. Its management depends on various factors and may involve medical management, surgical closure, or transcatheter intervention. Regular monitoring and follow-up are essential to ensure optimal outcomes and prevent complications.

Q 2. Discuss clinical features, pathophysiology, and management of cardiac tamponade. *(Refer Ques-2 Summer 2021-MUHS)*

Ans. Cardiac tamponade is a medical emergency characterized by the compression of the heart due to the accumulation of fluid or blood in the pericardial sac, leading to impaired cardiac function. Clinical features of cardiac tamponade can include:

- *Beck's triad:* This classic triad consists of:
    - *Hypotension:* Due to decreased cardiac output
    - *Jugular venous distension:* Elevated jugular venous pressure due to impaired venous return
    - *Muffled heart sounds:* Due to decreased transmission of heart sounds through the fluid-filled pericardial sac
- *Pulsus paradoxus*: A decrease in systolic blood pressure of >10 mm Hg during inspiration
- *Tachycardia:* Initially, the heart rate increases as a compensatory mechanism to maintain cardiac output.
- *Dyspnea:* Due to decreased cardiac output and impaired filling of the heart chambers

- *Chest pain:* Often described as sharp and pleuritic in nature but may not always be present.
- *Dizziness or syncope:* Due to decreased cerebral perfusion
- *Signs of shock:* Cold extremities, altered mental status, and reduced urine output may indicate severe cardiac tamponade.

Pathophysiology: Cardiac tamponade occurs when fluid accumulates in the pericardial sac, compressing the heart chambers and interfering with cardiac filling and function. This can result from various causes, including:
- *Pericardial effusion*: Accumulation of fluid in the pericardial space, which may occur due to inflammation (e.g., pericarditis), infection, malignancy, trauma, or iatrogenic causes (e.g., cardiac surgery and percutaneous interventions).
- *Rapid accumulation of fluid*: Acute tamponade can occur if fluid accumulates rapidly, leading to a sudden increase in intrapericardial pressure and compression of the heart.
- *Increased intrapericardial pressure*: Compression of the heart chambers reduces cardiac filling during diastole, leading to decreased volumes and cardiac output. This results in systemic hypoperfusion and the clinical manifestations of tamponade.

Management: The management of cardiac tamponade is aimed at relieving the compression on the heart and restoring cardiac function. Key interventions include:
- *Pericardiocentesis:* The immediate and definitive treatment for cardiac tamponade involves the insertion of a needle or catheter into the pericardial sac to drain the accumulated fluid. This procedure is often performed emergently at the bedside under echocardiographic guidance or in the operating room.
- *Pericardial window:* In cases of recurrent or persistent tamponade, a surgical procedure known as a pericardial window may be performed. This involves creating a permanent opening in the pericardium to allow for continuous drainage of fluid into the pleural space or abdomen.
- *Hemodynamic support:* Patients with severe cardiac tamponade may require hemodynamic support with IV fluids, vasopressors, or inotropic agents to maintain adequate perfusion until definitive treatment can be performed.
- *Underlying cause management:* Identifying and treating the underlying cause of pericardial effusion are essential to prevent recurrence of tamponade. This may involve addressing conditions such as pericarditis, infection, malignancy, or autoimmune diseases.
- *Close monitoring:* Patients with cardiac tamponade require close monitoring of vital signs, hemodynamic parameters, and cardiac

function to assess the response to treatment and detect any recurrence of tamponade.

In summary, cardiac tamponade is a life-threatening condition characterized by the compression of the heart due to the accumulation of fluid or blood in the pericardial sac. Prompt recognition and intervention, including pericardiocentesis and hemodynamic support, are essential for the management of cardiac tamponade and improving patient outcomes.

SHORT QUESTIONS AND ANSWERS

Q 1. Evaluation of Jones criteria. *(Refer 2021 MUHS)*

Ans. The Jones criteria are clinical criteria used to diagnose acute rheumatic fever (ARF), a systemic inflammatory condition that can occur following an untreated or inadequately treated group A streptococcal infection, most commonly streptococcal pharyngitis (strep throat). The criteria were first established in 1944 by T Duckett Jones and have since been revised multiple times to improve accuracy and specificity.

The Jones criteria are divided into two categories—(1) major criteria and (2) minor criteria. Diagnosis of ARF requires the presence of either two major criteria or one major criterion and two minor criteria, along with evidence of a preceding streptococcal infection. The criteria are as follows:

1. *Major criteria:*
   i. *Carditis:* Inflammation of the heart, typically involving the endocardium, myocardium, or pericardium. Manifestations may include tachycardia, new or changing heart murmurs, pericardial rubs, cardiomegaly, or evidence of congestive heart failure.
   ii. *Polyarthritis:* Acute migratory arthritis involving multiple large joints, often affecting the knees, ankles, elbows, and wrists. Joint pain and swelling may migrate from one joint to another over a period of days.
   iii. *Chorea:* Also known as Sydenham chorea, this is a characteristic movement disorder characterized by involuntary, purposeless movements, especially of the face and upper extremities. It may be accompanied by emotional lability, muscle weakness, and difficulty with fine motor tasks.
   iv. *Erythema marginatum:* A transient, nonpruritic rash characterized by pink, nonpruritic macules or papules with well-defined borders. The rash typically appears on the trunk and inner surfaces of the arms or thighs and may be exacerbated by heat or exercise.
   v. *Subcutaneous nodules:* Painful, firm, nontender nodules typically located over bony prominences or tendinous insertions, such as the extensor surfaces of the elbows, wrists, knees, or ankles.

2. *Minor criteria*:
    i. *Fever*: Elevated body temperature, although fever alone is not specific for ARF.
    ii. *Arthralgia*: Joint pain without objective signs of inflammation.
    iii. *Previous rheumatic fever or rheumatic heart disease*: History of ARF or rheumatic heart disease in the patient or first-degree relative.
    iv. *Elevated acute phase reactants*: Elevated erythrocyte sedimentation rate (ESR) or C-reactive protein (CRP) levels, indicating systemic inflammation.
    v. *Prolonged PR interval on ECG*: Evidence of conduction abnormalities, such as first-degree heart block, on electrocardiogram.

Evaluation and diagnosis: When evaluating a patient suspected of having ARF, healthcare providers must consider the patient's clinical presentation, history of streptococcal infection, and the presence of Jones criteria. Laboratory tests, including throat culture, rapid streptococcal antigen detection tests, and serological tests (anti-streptolysin O titer and anti-DNAse B titer), may also be performed to confirm recent streptococcal infection.

The diagnosis of ARF is primarily clinical, based on the presence of Jones Criteria and evidence of a preceding streptococcal infection. However, laboratory tests may aid in supporting the diagnosis and assessing disease severity. Treatment typically involves antibiotics to eradicate the underlying streptococcal infection, anti-inflammatory medications (e.g., aspirin and corticosteroids) to reduce inflammation and manage symptoms, and prophylactic antibiotics to prevent recurrent episodes of ARF and progression to rheumatic heart disease.

In summary, the Jones criteria are essential clinical guidelines used to diagnose ARF, a systemic inflammatory condition that can occur following untreated streptococcal infections. Evaluation involves assessing for the presence of major and minor criteria, along with evidence of a preceding streptococcal infection, and may also include laboratory tests to support the diagnosis and assess disease severity. Early recognition and treatment of ARF are critical to prevent complications such as rheumatic heart disease.

Q 2. Cyanotic spells.   *(Refer 2009/2014/2021 MUHS, 2009 MGR)*

Ans. Cyanotic spells, also known as cyanotic episodes or "tet spells," are acute exacerbations of cyanosis (bluish discoloration of the skin and mucous membranes) in infants and young children with congenital heart defects, particularly those with TOF. TOF is a complex congenital heart defect characterized by four main features:
1. *Ventricular septal defect (VSD):* A hole in the wall (septum) that separates the right and left ventricles.

2. *Pulmonary stenosis:* Narrowing of the pulmonary valve or pulmonary artery, which restricts blood flow to the lungs.
3. *Overriding aorta:* The aorta is positioned directly over the VSD, allowing oxygen-poor blood from the right ventricle to flow into the aorta and mix with oxygen-rich blood from the left ventricle.
4. *Right ventricular hypertrophy:* Enlargement of the right ventricle due to increased workload.

During a cyanotic spell, several factors contribute to a sudden decrease in systemic arterial oxygen saturation, leading to worsening cyanosis and potentially life-threatening hypoxemia. The exact mechanisms underlying cyanotic spells are not fully understood, but they are believed to involve a combination of increased right-to-left shunting of deoxygenated blood, decreased pulmonary blood flow, and increased systemic vascular resistance.

The typical triggers for cyanotic spells in infants and young children with TOF include:
- *Crying or agitation:* Increased sympathetic tone and increased oxygen demand can worsen right-to-left shunting and exacerbate cyanosis.
- *Feeding:* Increased oxygen demand during feeding can lead to decreased pulmonary blood flow and worsening cyanosis.
- *Exercise or exertion*: Physical activity can increase oxygen demand and worsen cyanosis.

Clinical manifestations of cyanotic spells may include:
- *Cyanosis:* Bluish discoloration of the skin, lips, and mucous membranes due to decreased oxygen saturation.
- *Respiratory distress:* Tachypnea (rapid breathing), dyspnea (shortness of breath), and respiratory distress may occur due to hypoxemia.
- *Irritability or agitation:* Infants may become fussy or irritable during cyanotic spells.
- *Syncope or loss of consciousness:* Severe hypoxemia can lead to loss of consciousness in some cases.

Management of cyanotic spells typically involves addressing the underlying cause (e.g., correcting dehydration and relieving airway obstruction) and providing supplemental oxygen to alleviate hypoxemia. In cases of severe cyanotic spells, interventions aimed at increasing systemic vascular resistance and reducing right-to-left shunting may be necessary. These interventions may include:
- *Knee-to-chest position*: Placing the child in a knee-to-chest position can increase systemic vascular resistance and improve pulmonary blood flow.
- *Oxygen therapy:* Administration of supplemental oxygen can alleviate hypoxemia and improve oxygen delivery to tissues.

- *IV fluids:* Administering IV fluids can help correct dehydration and increase intravascular volume, which may improve cardiac output and systemic perfusion.
- *Sedation:* Administering sedatives or analgesics may help calm the child and reduce agitation, thereby decreasing oxygen demand.

In severe cases refractory to medical management, emergency interventions such as IV morphine administration or even emergent surgical interventions to relieve obstruction (e.g., balloon valvuloplasty for pulmonary stenosis) may be necessary to stabilize the child and prevent further deterioration.

Overall, cyanotic spells are critical events in infants and children with congenital heart defects, particularly TOF, and require prompt recognition and appropriate management to prevent complications and optimize outcomes. Close monitoring and follow-up with a pediatric cardiologist are essential for infants and children with TOF to detect and manage cyanotic spells effectively.

Q 3. Stress echocardiography. *(Refer 2021 MUHS, 2016 MGR)*

Ans. Stress echocardiography is a diagnostic imaging technique that combines echocardiography (ultrasound imaging of the heart) with physical or pharmacological stress to evaluate cardiac function and blood flow under conditions of increased workload. It is commonly used to assess for ischemic heart disease, particularly in patients with suspected coronary artery disease (CAD) or to evaluate cardiac function in patients with known heart disease.

There are two main types of stress echocardiography:
1. *Exercise stress echocardiography:*
   i. During exercise stress echocardiography, the patient undergoes physical exercise, typically using a treadmill or stationary bicycle, to induce an increase in heart rate and workload.
   ii. Echocardiographic images are obtained before, during, and after exercise to assess changes in cardiac function, wall motion abnormalities, and myocardial perfusion.
   iii. Exercise stress echocardiography is useful for evaluating patients with suspected CAD, assessing functional capacity, determining the presence of exercise-induced ischemia, and assessing prognosis.
2. *Pharmacological stress echocardiography:*
   i. In cases where patients are unable to exercise or have contraindications to exercise, pharmacological agents are used to induce stress instead.
   ii. Common pharmacological stress agents include dobutamine (a β-adrenergic agonist), adenosine, and dipyridamole (vasodilators).

iii. Pharmacological stress echocardiography is particularly useful in patients with baseline ECG abnormalities, physical limitations, or other comorbidities that prevent them from exercising.
iv. Similar to exercise stress echocardiography, echocardiographic images are obtained before, during, and after stress to evaluate changes in cardiac function, wall motion abnormalities, and myocardial perfusion.

Indications for stress echocardiography include:
- *Evaluation of chest pain*: Assessing patients with chest pain or suspected angina to detect inducible myocardial ischemia.
- *Risk stratification*: Identifying patients at high risk for adverse cardiac events based on the presence of ischemia, left ventricular (LV) dysfunction, or other abnormalities.
- *Assessment of valvular heart disease*: Evaluating the hemodynamic significance and functional impact of valvular heart disease, such as aortic stenosis or mitral regurgitation.
- *Assessment of cardiomyopathy*: Evaluating cardiac function and wall motion abnormalities in patients with cardiomyopathy or heart failure.
- *Preoperative evaluation*: Assessing cardiac risk and functional capacity before noncardiac surgery, particularly in patients with known or suspected CAD.

Interpretation of stress echocardiography involves analyzing changes in wall motion abnormalities, LV function, and myocardial perfusion before and after stress. Inducible wall motion abnormalities or new perfusion defects observed during stress are suggestive of myocardial ischemia and may indicate underlying CAD.

Overall, stress echocardiography is a valuable noninvasive imaging modality for evaluating cardiac function, detecting ischemia, and guiding clinical decision-making in patients with known or suspected heart disease. It offers several advantages, including wide availability, real-time imaging capabilities, lack of radiation exposure, and ability to assess both anatomy and function simultaneously. However, it is important to recognize its limitations and potential pitfalls in interpretation, which may include image quality issues, technical challenges, and operator dependency. Close collaboration between clinicians and echocardiographers is essential to ensure accurate interpretation and appropriate clinical management based on the findings of stress echocardiography.

Q 4. S2 in health and disease.
(Refer 2014/2021 MUHS, 2019 Safdarjung)

Ans. The "S2" heart sound refers to the second heart sound, which is typically heard during cardiac auscultation and corresponds to the closure of the aortic and pulmonic valves. It consists of two components: A2 and P2. A2 represents the closure of the aortic valve, while P2 represents the closure of the pulmonic valve. Normally, the S2 heart sound is a crisp, high-pitched sound that occurs during early diastole.

In health: In a healthy individual, the S2 heart sound is typically normal in timing, intensity, and splitting. It is best heard at the base of the heart, specifically at the second intercostal space (right and left sternal borders), where the aortic and pulmonic valves are most audible.

Physiology of S2: During systole, the ventricles contract, causing a rise in pressure within the ventricles. As ventricular pressure exceeds aortic and pulmonic pressures, the aortic and pulmonic valves close, producing the A2 and P2 components of S2, respectively. The aortic valve typically closes slightly earlier than the pulmonic valve, resulting in a physiological split of the S2 sound. This splitting is more pronounced during inspiration due to changes in intrathoracic pressure.

Abnormalities and disease states:
- *Wide splitting of S2:* This can occur in conditions such as right bundle branch block (RBBB) or pulmonic stenosis, where delayed closure of the pulmonic valve prolongs the interval between A2 and P2, resulting in audible splitting throughout the respiratory cycle.
- *Fixed splitting of S2:* Seen in conditions such as ASD or VSD, where there is delayed closure of the pulmonic valve due to increased right ventricular volume. The split remains constant throughout the respiratory cycle.
- *Paradoxical splitting of S2:* Seen in conditions such as left bundle branch block (LBBB) or aortic stenosis, where there is delayed closure of the aortic valve due to prolonged LV contraction, leading to a reversal of the normal splitting pattern (P2-A2).
- *Single S2:* Occurs in conditions such as severe aortic stenosis or severe aortic regurgitation, where the aortic valve may not close properly, resulting in the absence of A2 and a single heart sound (single S2).

Clinical significance: Assessment of S2 characteristics and its variations plays a crucial role in diagnosing various cardiovascular conditions and guiding clinical management. Abnormalities in S2 can provide important diagnostic clues about underlying structural heart disease, valve abnormalities, or conduction disturbances. Careful auscultation and recognition of S2 abnormalities, along with other clinical findings and diagnostic tests, are essential for accurate diagnosis and appropriate management of cardiovascular conditions.

Q 5. Peripartum cardiomyopathy. *(Refer 2021 MUHS)*

Ans. Peripartum cardiomyopathy (PPCM) is a rare form of heart failure that occurs during the last month of pregnancy or within 5 months after giving birth (peripartum period) in women without a history of heart disease. It is characterized by the development of LV systolic dysfunction and heart failure symptoms, such as shortness of breath, fatigue, chest pain, and edema.

Epidemiology: PPCM affects approximately 1 in 1,000 to 1 in 4,000 pregnancies worldwide, but the incidence varies by region and ethnicity. Certain factors, such as advanced maternal age, multiparity (having multiple pregnancies), African descent, and certain genetic predispositions, may increase the risk of PPCM.

Pathophysiology: The exact cause of PPCM is not fully understood, but it is believed to involve a combination of genetic, hormonal, immunological, and environmental factors. Some proposed mechanisms include:
- *Cardiac remodeling:* Pregnancy-related hormonal changes and increased cardiac workload may lead to adverse remodeling of the heart, including dilation of the left ventricle and impairment of systolic function.
- *Inflammatory and immune factors:* Dysregulation of the immune system and inflammatory processes may contribute to myocardial damage and dysfunction.
- *Genetic predisposition:* Genetic factors may play a role in predisposing certain women to PPCM, although specific genetic mutations associated with the condition have not been clearly identified.
- *Nutritional deficiencies:* Inadequate intake of micronutrients such as selenium and coenzyme Q10, which are important for cardiac function, may contribute to the development of PPCM.

Clinical presentation: The clinical presentation of PPCM is similar to other forms of heart failure and may include symptoms such as:
- Shortness of breath (dyspnea), especially with exertion or lying flat
- Fatigue and weakness
- Swelling (edema) of the legs, ankles, or feet
- Palpitations or irregular heartbeats
- Chest pain or discomfort
- Decreased exercise tolerance
- Cough, especially at night
- Orthopnea (difficulty breathing while lying flat)

Diagnosis: Diagnosis of PPCM involves a thorough clinical evaluation, including medical history, physical examination, and diagnostic tests such as:

- *Echocardiography*: To assess LV function, chamber dimensions, and wall motion abnormalities.
- *Electrocardiogram (ECG)*: To evaluate heart rhythm and detect any conduction abnormalities.
- *Biomarkers*: Blood tests may show elevated levels of natriuretic peptides (BNP or NT-proBNP), indicating myocardial stress or heart failure.
- *Chest X-ray*: To assess for signs of pulmonary congestion or fluid accumulation in the lungs.

Management: The management of PPCM is aimed at improving symptoms, stabilizing cardiac function, and preventing complications. Treatment may include:
- *Medications*: Diuretics to reduce fluid overload, angiotensin-converting enzyme (ACE) inhibitors or angiotensin receptor blockers (ARBs) to improve cardiac function, beta-blockers to reduce heart rate and workload, and in certain cases, anticoagulants to prevent blood clots.
- *Supportive measures*: Rest, dietary modifications (low sodium intake), and close monitoring of fluid intake and output
- *Monitoring:* Regular follow-up with a cardiologist to assess cardiac function, adjust medications, and monitor for signs of worsening heart failure or complications.
- *Device therapy:* In severe cases, devices such as implantable cardioverter-defibrillators (ICDs) or cardiac resynchronization therapy (CRT) devices may be considered.
- *Pregnancy considerations*: Counseling regarding future pregnancies and contraceptive options, as subsequent pregnancies may increase the risk of recurrent PPCM.

Prognosis for PPCM varies depending on the severity of cardiac dysfunction and the response to treatment. While some women may experience complete recovery of cardiac function, others may develop chronic heart failure or require advanced therapies such as heart transplantation. Early recognition, prompt diagnosis, and appropriate management are essential for optimizing outcomes in women with PPCM.

Q 6. Recent guidelines of lipid management. *(Refer 2021 MUHS)*

Ans. Prominent guidelines for lipid management developed by the Association of Physicians of India (API). This guidance provides recommendations tailored to the Indian population and healthcare setting.

Key recommendations from the Indian Consensus Guidance on Management of Dyslipidemia include:
- *Risk stratification:* Similar to international guidelines, the Indian consensus guidance emphasizes the importance of risk stratification to

identify individuals at high risk for cardiovascular events. The guidance provides risk stratification tools specific to the Indian population.
- *Treatment goals:* The guidance recommends individualized treatment goals for lipid management based on the patient's cardiovascular risk profile. LDL cholesterol targets are provided based on risk categories, with lower targets for individuals at higher risk.
- *Lifestyle modifications:* Emphasis is placed on lifestyle modifications including dietary changes, regular physical activity, smoking cessation, and weight management as first-line therapy for dyslipidemia management. The guidance provides specific dietary recommendations tailored to the Indian diet.
- *Pharmacological therapy:* Pharmacological therapy with statins is recommended for patients who do not achieve lipid targets with lifestyle modifications alone. The choice of statin and intensity of therapy depend on the patient's cardiovascular risk profile and lipid levels.
- *Combination therapy:* The guidance discusses the use of combination therapy with statins and other lipid-lowering agents (e.g., ezetimibe) for patients who require additional LDL cholesterol reduction despite maximally tolerated statin therapy.
- *Monitoring and follow-up:* Recommendations are provided for monitoring lipid levels and assessing treatment response over time. Regular follow-up visits are recommended to assess adherence to therapy, monitor for adverse effects, and adjust treatment as needed.

It is important to note that guidelines may vary among different professional organizations and may be updated periodically based on new evidence. Healthcare providers in India should refer to the most recent guidelines from reputable sources such as the Association of Physicians of India or other relevant professional organizations for the latest recommendations on lipid management tailored to the Indian population.

SUGGESTED READING

1. Adler Y, Ristić AD, Imazio M, Brucato A, Pankuweit S, Burazor I, et al. Cardiac tamponade. Nat Rev Dis Primers. 2023;9(1):1-18.
2. Badla O, Goit R, Saddik SE, Dawood S, Rabih AM, Mohammed A, et al. The Multidisciplinary Management of Perianal Fistulas in Crohn's Disease: A Systematic Review. Cureus. 2022;14(9):e29347.
3. Basnet B, Adhikari G. (2023). Exploring Pulmonary Embolism-Causes, Symptoms, And Effective Treatment. [online] Available from https://ehealthyinfo.com/blog/pulmonary-embolism-symptoms-causes-treatment/ [Last accessed April, 2024].
4. Britannica. (2024). Childhood Diseases & Disorders Browse-Page 1. [online] Available from https://www.britannica.com/browse/Childhood-Diseases-Disorders/1 [Last accessed April, 2024].

5. Chen Y, Huai-zhong MU. Natural resources, carbon trading policies and total factor carbon efficiency: A new direction for China's economy. Res Policy. 2023;86:104183.
6. Coppi F, Bucciarelli V, Solodka K, Selleri V, Zanini G, Pinti M, et al. The Impact of Stress and Social Determinants on Diet in Cardiovascular Prevention in Young Women. Nutrients. 2024;16(7):1044.
7. Debbal SM. Computerized Heart Sounds Analysis. [online] Available from: https://www.intechopen.com/chapters/19510 [Last accessed April, 2024].
8. Dokumen.pub. (2021). Oxford Textbook of Pediatric Pain [2 ed]. [online] Available from https://dokumen.pub/oxford-textbook-of-pediatric-pain-2nbsped-0198818769-9780198818762-m-7077649.html [Last accessed April, 2024].
9. Fukuda Y, Uchida Y, Ando K, Manabe R, Tanaka A, Sagara H. Risk factors for interstitial lung disease in patients with non-small cell lung cancer with epidermal growth factor receptor-tyrosine kinase inhibitors: A systematic review and meta-analysis. Respir Investig. 2024;62(3):481-7.
10. Humphrey A, Carapetis J, Remenyi B. Acute Rheumatic Fever and Chronic Rheumatic Disease. Philadelphia: Springer eBooks. 2023.
11. Ka G. Perspectives on intra-aortic balloon-pump timing. Crit Care Nurs Clin North Am. 1989;1(3):469-74.
12. Kohlman-Trigoboff D. Review of article: Inclisiran for the treatment of heterozygous familial hypercholesterolemia. N Engl J Med. 2020;382:1520-30.
13. Lazea C. (2017). Emergency Pericardiocentesis in Children. [online] Available from: https://www.intechopen.com/chapters/57490 [Last accessed April, 2024].
14. Pulsenotes. (2024). Cardiac tamponade. [online] Available from https://app.pulsenotes.com/medicine/cardiology/notes/cardiac-tamponade [Last accessed April, 2024].
15. Visser KR, Mook GA, van der Wall E, Zijlstra WG. Theory of the determination of systolic time intervals by impedance cardiography. Biol Psychol. 1993;36(1-2):43-50.

DM CARDIOLOGY EXAMINATION

Paper 1 (Set 4)

LONG-ESSAY QUESTIONS AND ANSWERS

Q 1. Discuss congenital abnormalities of the tricuspid valve.
(Refer 2015/2022-MUHS)

Ans. Congenital abnormalities of the tricuspid valve represent a diverse spectrum of structural defects that can significantly impact cardiac function and overall health. The tricuspid valve, situated between the right atrium and the right ventricle of the heart, plays a crucial role in facilitating the unidirectional flow of blood during the cardiac cycle. Any malformation or dysfunction of this valve can lead to a variety of clinical manifestations, ranging from asymptomatic to life-threatening. In this essay, we will explore the different types of congenital abnormalities of the tricuspid valve, their pathophysiology, clinical presentations, diagnostic approaches, and management strategies.

One of the rarest congenital abnormalities affecting the tricuspid valve is tricuspid valve atresia. In this condition, the tricuspid valve is either absent or severely underdeveloped, leading to a complete obstruction of blood flow from the right atrium to the right ventricle. As a result, affected individuals typically present with cyanosis and signs of right heart failure shortly after birth. Tricuspid valve atresia is often associated with other cardiac defects, such as ventricular septal defects (VSDs) or hypoplastic right ventricle, and requires prompt surgical intervention to establish adequate pulmonary blood flow.

Tricuspid valve stenosis is another congenital anomaly characterized by narrowing of the tricuspid valve orifice, resulting in obstructed blood flow from the right atrium to the right ventricle. The narrowing may be due to abnormal valve leaflet formation, fusion of valve cusps, or thickening of the valve apparatus. Patients with tricuspid stenosis typically present with symptoms of right heart failure, including fatigue, hepatomegaly, and peripheral edema. Diagnosis is confirmed through echocardiography, which demonstrates decreased valve orifice area and elevated right atrial pressures. Treatment options may include balloon valvuloplasty or surgical repair, depending on the severity of the stenosis.

Ebstein's anomaly is a rare congenital heart defect characterized by abnormal displacement of the septal and posterior leaflets of the tricuspid valve toward the apex of the right ventricle. This results in an "atrialized" portion of the right ventricle, which has reduced contractile function.

Patients with Ebstein's anomaly may present with a wide range of symptoms, including cyanosis, palpitations, and exercise intolerance. Diagnosis is typically made based on echocardiographic findings, which demonstrate the abnormal positioning of the tricuspid valve leaflets. Management of Ebstein's anomaly may involve medical therapy to alleviate symptoms and surgical repair to improve valve function and restore cardiac anatomy.

Tricuspid valve regurgitation occurs when the valve leaflets fail to close properly during systole, allowing blood to leak backward from the right ventricle into the right atrium. Congenital causes of tricuspid regurgitation may include abnormalities in valve leaflet formation or malformation of the chordae tendineae. Patients with tricuspid regurgitation may present with symptoms such as fatigue, exertional dyspnea, and peripheral edema. Diagnosis is confirmed through echocardiography, which demonstrates the presence of regurgitant flow across the tricuspid valve. Management options for tricuspid regurgitation may include medical therapy to alleviate symptoms and surgical repair or replacement of the valve in severe cases.

Tricuspid valve dysplasia refers to abnormal development of the tricuspid valve leaflets, chordae tendineae, or papillary muscles. This can result in a spectrum of abnormalities ranging from mild thickening of the valve leaflets to more severe deformities that impair valve function. Tricuspid valve dysplasia may predispose individuals to tricuspid regurgitation or stenosis and often requires surgical intervention for correction.

In conclusion, congenital abnormalities of the tricuspid valve represent a diverse array of structural defects that can have significant implications for cardiac function and overall health. Early recognition and appropriate management of these anomalies are essential for optimizing outcomes and improving the quality of life for affected individuals. A multidisciplinary approach involving pediatric cardiologists, cardiac surgeons, and other healthcare providers is often necessary to provide comprehensive care for patients with congenital tricuspid valve abnormalities. Through advances in diagnostic techniques and surgical interventions, the prognosis for individuals with these conditions continues to improve, offering hope for a better future.

Q 2. Describe embryogenesis of interatrial septum. Describe embryological basis for all types of septal defects. *(Refer 2022 MUHS)*

Ans. The embryogenesis of the interatrial septum, which forms the basis for atrial septal defects (ASDs), involves complex developmental processes during fetal development. Understanding these processes is crucial for comprehending the various types of ASDs and their clinical implications. Let's delve into the embryological journey of the interatrial septum and its relevance to ASDs.

Embryogenesis of the Interatrial Septum
During early fetal development, the heart begins as a simple tube composed of myocardial cells. As development progresses, the heart undergoes intricate morphological changes, including the formation of septa that partition the heart into distinct chambers.

Formation of the Septum Primum
Initially, a crescent-shaped ridge known as the septum primum forms in the primitive atrium, protruding toward the endocardial cushion located between the atria.

This structure gradually elongates downward, partially dividing the primitive atrium into left and right portions. However, an opening known as the ostium primum persists at the lower end of the septum primum.

Development of the Foramen Primum
As the septum primum elongates, it creates a temporary opening called the foramen primum, allowing blood to pass from the right to the left atrium.

Formation of the Septum Secundum
Concurrently, another crescent-shaped ridge, the septum secundum, develops on the right side of the atrial cavity, adjacent to the septum primum.

Unlike the septum primum, the septum secundum does not completely fuse with the endocardial cushion, leaving an opening called the foramen ovale.

Closure of the Foramen Ovale
As fetal circulation transitions from the placental to pulmonary circulation after birth, changes in pressure gradients and oxygenation prompt the functional closure of the foramen ovale.

Eventually, the septum primum and septum secundum fuse to form the mature interatrial septum, separating the left and right atria.

Embryological Basis for Arterial Septal Defects
Arterial septal defects arise from abnormalities in the formation of the interatrial septum during embryogenesis. These defects result in abnormal communication between the left and right atria, leading to shunting of blood and potential hemodynamic consequences. Here are the embryological bases for the various types of ASDs:
- *Secundum ASD:*
  - Secundum ASD is the most common type of ASD and typically results from incomplete fusion of the septum primum and septum secundum during fetal development.
  - Failure of the septum primum and septum secundum to fuse completely leads to a persistent opening in the interatrial septum, allowing left-to-right shunting of blood.

- *Primum ASD:*
  - Primum ASD, also known as atrioventricular septal defect (AVSD), occurs due to incomplete fusion of the endocardial cushion during embryogenesis.
  - This defect is often associated with abnormalities in the AV valves and is frequently seen in individuals with Down syndrome.
- *Sinus venosus ASD:*
  - Sinus venosus ASD results from an abnormal connection between the superior or inferior vena cava and the right atrium, near the entrance of the superior vena cava.
  - It arises due to incomplete development of the septum secundum or displacement of the septum primum toward the superior vena cava.
- *Coronary sinus ASD*:
  - Coronary sinus ASD involves an abnormal communication between the coronary sinus and the left atrium.
  - It occurs due to defects in the development of the septum secundum or the tissue surrounding the coronary sinus.

In summary, the embryogenesis of the interatrial septum is a complex process that lays the foundation for the formation of ASDs. Abnormalities in this developmental process can lead to various types of ASDs, each with distinct anatomical features and clinical implications. Understanding the embryological basis of these defects is essential for accurate diagnosis and appropriate management of affected individuals.

SHORT QUESTIONS AND ANSWERS

Q 1. Scimitar syndrome. *(Refer 2022 MUHS, 2012/2019/2024 MGR)*

Ans. Scimitar syndrome, also known as congenital pulmonary venolobar syndrome, is a rare congenital anomaly characterized by a combination of cardiovascular and pulmonary abnormalities. The syndrome derives its name from the resemblance of the anomalous pulmonary vein to a curved Turkish sword, known as a scimitar. Here, we'll delve into the key features, etiology, clinical manifestations, diagnosis, and management of Scimitar syndrome.

Features
- *Anomalous pulmonary vein:* The hallmark feature of Scimitar syndrome is the anomalous pulmonary vein, typically the right pulmonary vein, which drains into the inferior vena cava (IVC) or one of its tributaries rather than the left atrium.

- *Pulmonary hypoplasia:* Affected individuals often present with varying degrees of hypoplasia or underdevelopment of the right lung due to reduced blood flow and aeration.
- *Cardiac anomalies:* Scimitar syndrome may be associated with other cardiac anomalies, including ASDs, VSDs, PDA, and anomalies of the AV valves.

Etiology

The exact cause of Scimitar syndrome remains unclear. It is believed to result from abnormal development of the pulmonary venous system during embryogenesis.

Genetic factors may play a role, as Scimitar syndrome has been reported in families with a history of congenital heart defects.

Clinical Manifestations

Clinical presentation varies depending on the severity of pulmonary hypoplasia and associated cardiac anomalies.

Infants may present with respiratory distress, cyanosis, failure to thrive, and recurrent respiratory infections.

Older children and adults may remain asymptomatic or present with symptoms related to pulmonary hypertension or cardiac arrhythmias.

Diagnosis

Diagnosis of Scimitar syndrome is typically made through a combination of clinical evaluation, imaging studies, and cardiac catheterization.

Chest X-ray may reveal an abnormal shadow resembling a scimitar, indicating the anomalous pulmonary vein.

Echocardiography can confirm the presence of the anomalous pulmonary vein and associated cardiac anomalies.

Cardiac MRI or CT angiography provides detailed anatomical information and helps assess the extent of pulmonary hypoplasia.

Management

Treatment of Scimitar syndrome depends on the severity of symptoms and associated anomalies.

Surgical intervention may be necessary to repair cardiac defects, reroute the anomalous pulmonary vein to the left atrium, and improve lung perfusion.

Patients with mild symptoms and minimal pulmonary hypoplasia may require conservative management with close monitoring.

In conclusion, Scimitar syndrome is a rare congenital anomaly characterized by anomalous pulmonary venous drainage, pulmonary hypoplasia, and associated cardiac defects. Early diagnosis and appropriate management are essential to optimize outcomes and improve the quality of life for affected individuals. Further research into the underlying etiology and genetic factors may provide valuable insights into the pathogenesis of this intriguing condition.

Q 2. Fate of the left and right ventricle after TOF repair.
(Refer 2022 MUHS)

Ans. Following surgical repair of Tetralogy of Fallot (TOF), the left and right ventricles undergo distinct changes that are essential to understand for comprehensive patient management.

Left Ventricle
Prior to repair, the left ventricle in TOF patients may be relatively small and underdeveloped due to reduced blood flow from the right ventricular outflow obstruction.

After surgical correction, the left ventricle may gradually remodel and hypertrophy over time. This adaptation is crucial as it helps the left ventricle to accommodate systemic pressures efficiently.

Regular monitoring of LV function through echocardiography is essential postrepair to detect any signs of dysfunction or inadequate hypertrophy.

Right Ventricle
The right ventricle bears the brunt of the workload in TOF patients due to the primary defect in the right ventricular outflow tract.

Surgical repair aims to relieve obstructions and restore pulmonary blood flow, alleviating the strain on the right ventricle.

Despite repair, the right ventricle may still exhibit some degree of residual dysfunction or dilation, particularly if there were significant pre-existing abnormalities.

Long-term follow-up is crucial to monitor right ventricular function and detect any signs of deterioration, such as right ventricular dilation, reduced contractility, or arrhythmias.

In summary, understanding the fate of the left and right ventricles after TOF repair is vital for optimizing patient care. Close monitoring of ventricular function through imaging modalities and regular follow-up visits are essential components of long-term management strategies.

Q 3. Lipoprotein A. *(Refer 2022 MUHS, 2012 MGR)*

Ans. Lipoprotein(A), often abbreviated as Lp(a), is a lipoprotein particle that has been increasingly recognized for its significant role in cardiovascular health. Comprising of a cholesterol-rich core and a protein called apolipoprotein(a), Lp(a) is similar in structure to low-density lipoprotein (LDL) but has an additional protein component.

Lp(a) has garnered attention due to its association with an increased risk of cardiovascular disease, including coronary artery disease, stroke, and peripheral arterial disease. Elevated levels of Lp(a) have been identified as an independent risk factor for these conditions, with higher levels correlating with a greater risk.

Despite its importance, Lp(a) is not routinely measured in standard lipid panels. However, its measurement may be warranted in individuals with a family history of premature cardiovascular disease or those who have recurrent cardiovascular events despite optimal management of traditional risk factors.

Currently, there are limited therapeutic options specifically targeting Lp(a). However, ongoing research is exploring various strategies, including antisense oligonucleotide therapy and monoclonal antibodies, to lower Lp(a) levels and potentially reduce cardiovascular risk.

Given its emerging significance, understanding and monitoring Lp(a) levels can provide valuable insights into an individual's cardiovascular risk profile, enabling more targeted approaches to prevention and management.

Q 4. Dynamic auscultation. *(Refer 2022 MUHS, 2015 MGR)*

Ans. Dynamic auscultation is a crucial technique utilized in clinical cardiology for a more comprehensive assessment of cardiac function and pathology. This approach involves listening to heart sounds and murmurs while manipulating various patient factors such as position, respiration, and physiological maneuvers. By incorporating dynamic changes, clinicians can glean additional information beyond what is typically observed during a static examination.

During dynamic auscultation, several maneuvers may be employed, including:

- *Altering patient position:* Patients may be asked to sit up, lie down, or shift to a left lateral decubitus position. These positional changes can affect the distribution of blood flow and the intensity of murmurs, aiding in the diagnosis of certain conditions like mitral valve prolapse or aortic regurgitation.
- *Physiological maneuvers:* Patients may be instructed to perform actions such as the Valsalva maneuver, squatting, or standing. These maneuvers influence factors such as preload, afterload, and intrathoracic pressure, leading to changes in the intensity and timing of heart sounds and murmurs. For instance, the intensity of hypertrophic obstructive cardiomyopathy murmurs may vary with maneuvers like the Valsalva maneuver or standing.

- *Respiratory variations:* Observing how heart sounds and murmurs change with different phases of respiration can provide insights into conditions such as constrictive pericarditis or cardiac tamponade.

Dynamic auscultation aids in the diagnosis and assessment of various cardiac conditions, including valvular disorders, congenital heart diseases, and cardiomyopathies. By evaluating how heart sounds and murmurs respond to dynamic changes, clinicians can better determine the severity of pathology, differentiate between innocent and pathological murmurs, and guide treatment decisions.

In clinical practice, dynamic auscultation complements traditional static auscultation, enhancing the diagnostic accuracy and clinical evaluation of cardiovascular patients. It is an indispensable tool in the armamentarium of cardiologists, enabling a more thorough understanding of cardiac physiology and pathology.

Q 5. Conduction system pacing. *(Refer 2022 MUHS)*

Ans. Conduction system pacing is a specialized technique used in the field of cardiology to optimize cardiac pacing therapy by directly stimulating the heart's native conduction system. Unlike traditional pacing methods that involve stimulating the myocardium, conduction system pacing targets-specific regions of the heart's intrinsic conduction system, such as the His bundle or the left bundle branch, to achieve more physiological pacing.

This approach offers several advantages over conventional pacing methods:
- *Physiological pacing:* By targeting the native conduction system, conduction system pacing mimics the heart's natural electrical activation pattern, resulting in more synchronized and coordinated ventricular activation. This can potentially improve hemodynamics and reduce the risk of pacing-induced cardiomyopathy.
- *Preservation of AV synchrony:* Conduction system pacing maintains the normal sequence of atrial and ventricular activation, preserving AV synchrony and avoiding the adverse effects associated with ventricular pacing.
- *Lower risk of heart failure progression:* Studies have suggested that conduction system pacing may be associated with a lower risk of heart failure hospitalization and mortality compared to traditional right ventricular pacing, particularly in patients with heart failure and reduced ejection fraction.

Conduction system pacing can be achieved using different techniques, including:
- *His bundle pacing:* Directly pacing the His bundle or the bundle of His, which is located in the interventricular septum.

- *Left bundle branch pacing:* Stimulating the left bundle branch to achieve ventricular activation.

Despite its potential benefits, conduction system pacing requires specialized equipment, expertise, and careful patient selection. Factors such as anatomical variations, lead positioning, and pacing thresholds need to be considered to ensure optimal outcomes.

In summary, conduction system pacing represents a promising advancement in cardiac pacing therapy, offering more physiological pacing and potential benefits in terms of hemodynamics and clinical outcomes. As cardiologists, understanding and incorporating this technique into our practice can help optimize patient care and improve long-term outcomes for individuals requiring pacing therapy.

Q 6. Jugular venous pressure waveforms in health and disease.
(Refer 2022 MUHS, 2014/2020 Safdarjung)

Ans. Understanding JVP waveforms is crucial for assessing cardiac function and diagnosing various cardiovascular conditions. In both health and disease, changes in JVP waveforms provide valuable insights into hemodynamics and cardiac performance.

In health:
- *Normal JVP waveform:* In healthy individuals, the JVP waveform typically exhibits three positive waves (a, c, and v) and two descents (x and y).
  - The "a" wave corresponds to atrial contraction and is seen as a small upward deflection in the JVP waveform.
  - The "c" wave represents the bulging of the tricuspid valve into the right atrium during ventricular systole, causing a slight elevation in JVP.
  - The "v" wave occurs during ventricular filling and corresponds to the rise in JVP as blood flows into the right atrium.
  - The "x" descent follows the "c" wave and represents atrial relaxation and ventricular filling.
  - The "y" descent occurs as the tricuspid valve opens, allowing blood to flow from the right atrium to the right ventricle, resulting in a decline in JVP.

In disease:
- *Elevated JVP:* Conditions such as right-sided heart failure, tricuspid regurgitation, constrictive pericarditis, and pulmonary hypertension can lead to elevated JVP. In these cases, the JVP waveform may show prominent "a" and "v" waves with diminished "x" and "y" descents.
  - *Absent "a" wave:* Atrial fibrillation or atrial flutter can result in the loss of the "a" wave, leading to a flat JVP waveform.

- *Cannon "a" wave:* In conditions with AV dissociation, such as complete heart block, a prominent "a" wave may be observed in the JVP waveform due to atrial contraction against a closed tricuspid valve.
- *Kussmaul sign:* In conditions like constrictive pericarditis or restrictive cardiomyopathy, impaired ventricular filling results in an exaggerated "y" descent and a steep "x" descent, known as Kussmaul sign.
- *Absent "x" and "y" descents:* In conditions such as tricuspid stenosis or severe right ventricular dysfunction, the "x" and "y" descents may be absent, resulting in a "square root sign" appearance of the JVP waveform.

In summary, interpreting JVP waveforms is a valuable skill for cardiologists, aiding in the diagnosis and management of various cardiovascular conditions. By understanding the characteristic changes in JVP waveforms in health and disease, clinicians can better assess cardiac function and hemodynamics in their patients.

SUGGESTED READING

1. Abdulla R. Heart Diseases in Children—A Pediatrician's Guide. Philadelphia: New York, NY: Springer Nature; 2011.
2. Badano LP, Lang RM, Muraru D. Textbook of Three-Dimensional Echocardiography. Cham: Springer International Publishing; 2019.
3. EPDF. (2024). Congenital Heart Defects. Decision Making for Surgery: Volume 3: CT-Scan and MRI (Congenital Heart Defects: Decision Making for Surgery). [online]. Available from: https://epdf.tips/congenital-heart-defects-decision-making-for-surgery-volume-3-ct-scan-and-mri-co.html [Last accessed May, 2024].
4. Freedom RM, Yoo SJ, Mikailian H, Williams WG. The Natural and Modified History of Congenital Heart Disease. New Jersey: Wiley Books. 2003.
5. Iannuzzo G, Tripaldella M, Mallardo V, Morgillo ME, Vitelli N, Iannuzzi A, et al. Lipoprotein(a) Where Do We Stand? From the Physiopathology to Innovative Terapy. Biomedicines. 2021;9(7):838-8.
6. Lai CH, Wu JM, Yang YJ. Ebstein's Anomaly of the Tricuspid Valve in Combination of Tetralogy of Fallot: Total Correction in Infancy. Ann Thorac Surg. 2007;83(1):304-6.
7. Nihoyannopoulos P, Kisslo J. Echocardiography. Cham: Springer International Publishing; 2018.
8. Seward JB. Ebstein's Anomaly: Echocardiography. 1993;10(6):641-64.
9. Sinju KR, Bhangare BB, Prakash J, Debnath AK, NS Ramgir. Effect of ZnO morphologies on its sensor response and corresponding E-nose performance. Solid-state Mat Adv Technol. 2023;298:116870.
10. Sisini F, Tessari M, Gadda G, Domenico GD, Taibi A, Menegatti E, et al. An Ultrasonographic Technique to Assess the Jugular Venous Pulse: A Proof of Concept. Ultrasound Med Biol. 2015;41(5):1334-41.

11. Skeete J, Huang HD, Mazur A, Sharma PS, Englestein E, Trohman RG, et al. Evolving Concepts in Cardiac Physiologic Pacing in the Era of Conduction System Pacing. Am J Cardiol. 2024;212:51-66.
12. Wong PC, Miller-Hance WC. Transesophageal Echocardiography for Congenital Heart Disease. Philadelphia: Springer Nature; 2014.
13. Wong PC, Miller-Hance WC. Transesophageal Echocardiography for Congenital Heart Disease. Philadelphia: Springer Nature; 2014.
14. Yardley R, Nelson G. Central venous and pulmonary artery catheters. Anaesth Intensive Care Med. 2023;24(12):781-4.

Index

A

Acute coronary syndromes 23
Adenosine 3, 37
Agitation 5, 36
Alkalosis 27
Ankle brachial index 12
    calculation of 12
Anomalous pulmonary vein 47, 48
Antibiotic
    therapy 20
    use, prior 19
Aorta, overriding 4, 36
Aortitis 25
    diagnosis of 25
Apolipoprotein 49
Arrhythmias 11
    treatment of 2, 3
Arterial septal defects, embryological basis for 46
Arthralgia 35
Athlete's heart 8, 10
    distinguishing 9
    management of 10
Atrial arrhythmias 16
Atrial septal defects 45
    classification of 15
    description of 15
    pathophysiology of 16
    primum 16, 47
    types of 15
Atrioventricular node 18
    location of 21
Atrioventricular reentrant tachycardia 3
Atrioventricular synchrony, preservation of 51
Autoimmune aortitis 25

B

Bartonella 19
Beck's triad 32
Blood
    pressure measurement 12
    viscosity 21
    supply 18, 29
Bradycardia 9
Breath 5
Breathing, rapid 5
Bundle branches 18
Bundle of His 18

C

Cardiac abnormalities 4
Cardiac anomalies 48
Cardiac conduction system 18
Cardiac dimensions, increased 9
Cardiac failure 16
Cardiac function, normal 9
Cardiac hypertrophy 9
Cardiac remodeling 40
Cardiac tamponade
    management of 32
    pathophysiology of 32
Cardiomyopathy, assessment of 38
Cardiovascular conditions, management of 39
Cardiovascular symptoms 27
Carditis 34
Cataracts 27
    development of 27
Catheter ablation 3
Central venous pressure 8
Chamber dimensions 28
Chest pain 33
    evaluation of 38
Chordae tendineae 45
Chorea 34
Chronic kidney disease 27
Combination therapy 42
Conduction system pacing 51
Congenital heart
    defect 31
    disease 22
Conotruncal abnormality, management of 1
Consciousness, loss of 5, 36
Coronary sinus atrial septal defect 16, 47
Coxiella burnetii 19
Crying 5
Culture negative endocarditis 19
Cyanosis 2, 5, 36
Cyanotic spell 4, 6, 35
    clinical manifestations of 5
    management of 5, 36

D

Dermatological manifestations 27
Device therapy 11, 41
Digital ulcers 6
Dipyridamole 37
Disease severity, assessment of 13
Dizziness 33
Dynamic auscultation 50
Dyspnea 5, 32

E

Ebstein's anomaly 44
Echocardiography 41
Electrical cardioversion 3
Electrocardiogram 41
Electrocardiographic changes 9
Embryology 1, 31
Empirical therapy 20
Endothelial cells 6
Endothelial receptor
    antagonists 6
    types of 6
Endothelin release 17
Enhanced cardiac function 9
Erythema marginatum 34
Exercise 5, 36
    stress echocardiography 37
Exertion 5, 36
Exertional dyspnea 45

F

Factors influencing pulmonary vascular
    resistance 21
Fastidious organisms 19
Fatigue, fate of 45
Feeding 5
Fever 35
Fibrous cap, thin 22
Fluid, rapid accumulation of 33
Foramen
    ovale, closure of 46
    primum, development of 46

G

Genetic counseling 2
Genetic predisposition 40
Great arteries, transposition of 1

H

Heart
    muscle 7
    right ventricle of 44
Heart failure 2, 8, 11
    progression, lower risk of 51
    right-sided 16
Hemodynamic support 33
His bundle pacing 51
Hypertrophic obstructive cardiomyopathy
    murmurs 50
Hypertrophy 10
Hypocalcemia 27
    chronic 27
    treatment of 28
Hypomagnesemia 27
Hypoparathyroidism 27
Hypotension 32

I

Iatrogenic causes 33
Idiopathic aortitis 25
    management of 26
Immune factors 40
Implantable cardioverter-defibrillators 11
Infection 33
Infectious aortitis 25
Inflammation 22
Inflammatory factors 40
Interatrial septum
    development of 15
    embryogenesis of 46
Intraoperative management 8
Intrapericardial pressure, increased 33
Irritability 5, 36
Ischemic stroke 23

J

Jones criteria, evaluation of 34
Jugular venous
    distension 32
    pressure waveforms 52

K

Kent bundles 3
Knee-to-chest position 5, 36
Koch's triangle 20, 21
    anatomy of 20
    septal border of 20
Kussmaul sign 53

L

Left bundle branch pacing 52
Left ventricle 49
   anatomy of 28
   fate of 49
Left ventricular remodeling 10
Lifestyle modifications 12, 42
Lipid management, recent guidelines of 41
Lipid-rich core 23
Lipoprotein
   A 49
   low-density 49

M

Mahaim fibers 3
Malignancy 33
Medical management 32
Medical stabilization 2
Medications 27, 41
Microbial characteristics 19
Muffled heart sounds 32
Myocardial contractility 7
Myocardium 7

N

Natriuretic peptides release 17
Neovascularization 23
Neurohormonal activation 11
Neurohumoral mechanisms 16
Neurological symptoms 27
Neuromuscular symptoms 27
Nonfunctional fetal lungs 31
Nutritional deficiencies 40

O

Oxygen therapy 5, 36

P

Pancreatitis, acute 27
Papillary muscles 29
Paradoxical embolism 16
Patent ductus arteriosus 31
   classification of 31
   management of 31
   pathophysiology of 31
Pericardial effusion 33
Pericardial window 33
Pericardiocentesis 33
Pericarditis 33
Peripartum cardiomyopathy 40
Peripheral arterial disease diagnosis 13
Peripheral edema 45
Persistent truncus arteriosus 1
Pharmacological stress
   echocardiography 37
Pharmacological therapy 11, 42
Physiological pacing 51
Plaque
   erosion 23
   rupture 23
Polyarthritis 34
P-pulmonale 26
Primum septa 15
Prostacyclin receptor antagonists 7
Pulmonary arterial hypertension 6, 7
Pulmonary arteries 21
   wedge pressure 8
Pulmonary arteriolar tone 21
Pulmonary hypertension 16, 21
Pulmonary hypoplasia 48
Pulmonary stenosis 1, 4, 36
Pulmonary vascular resistance 21
   measurement of 22
Pulsus paradoxus 32

R

Radiofrequency catheter ablation 3
Renin-angiotensin-aldosterone system
   activation 17
Respiratory
   disorders 22
   variations 51
   distress 2, 5, 36
Rheumatic fever, previous 35
Rheumatic heart disease 35
Right bundle branch block
   complete 26
   incomplete 26
Right ventricle 49
Right ventricular
   hypertrophy 5, 26, 36
   outflow tract 1

S

Scimitar syndrome 47, 48
   cause of 48
   diagnosis of 48
   treatment of 48
Secundum atrial septal defects 15
Secundum septa 15

Sedation 5, 37
Septal defects, types of 45
Septum primum, formation of 46
Septum secundum, formation of 46
Serum calcium 28
Shock, signs of 33
Shortness 5
Sinoatrial node 18
Sinus venosus atrial septal defects 16, 47
Starling's law 7, 8
Stenosis 45
Stress echocardiography 37
 types of 37
Stroke volume 7
Subcutaneous nodules 34
Supportive measures 41
Supraventricular tachyarrhythmias 4
Sydenham chorea 34
Sympathetic nervous system activation 16
Symptomatic arrhythmias, acute
 management of 3, 4
Syncope 5, 33, 36
Systemic sclerosis 6

T

Tachycardia 32
Tachypnea 5
Tetralogy of Fallot 1
Ticagrelor 23
Transcatheter closure 32
Trauma 33
Tricuspid regurgitation 45
 congenital causes of 45
Tricuspid stenosis 44
Tricuspid valve
 congenital abnormalities of 44
 dysplasia 45
 regurgitation 45
 stenosis 44
T-wave changes 26

U

Underlying cause management 33

V

Vagal maneuvers 3
Valves 29
Valvular heart disease, assessment of 38
Vasodilators 37
Venous return 7
Ventricular dilatation 10
Ventricular function, altered 11
Ventricular geometry, changes in 10
Ventricular septal defect 4, 35, 44
Vitamin D
 deficiency 27, 28
 supplementation 28
Vulnerable plaque, pathology of 22

W

Wall thickness 28
Wolff-Parkinson-White syndrome 2

EU GSPR Authorised Reprsentative
Logos Europe, 9 rue Nicolas Poussin
1700, La Rochelle, France
Phone: +33 (0) 6 67 93 73 78
E-mail: contact@logoseurope.eu

www.ingramcontent.com/pod-product-compliance
Ingram Content Group UK Ltd.
Pitfield, Milton Keynes, MK11 3LW, UK
UKHW050455150426
5217IPUK00025B/1690